DISINFECTION

Edited by **Sahra Kırmusaoğlu**

Disinfection
http://dx.doi.org/10.5772/intechopen.71513
Edited by Sahra Kırmusaoğlu

Contributors

Raymond Nims, S. Steve Zhou, Cameron Wilde, Zheng Chen, Tanya Kapes, Jennifer Purgill, Donna Suchmann, Tatiana Hruskova, Naďa Sasáková, Gabriela Gregová, Zuzana Bujdošová, Ingrid Papajová, Milton Rosero Moreano, Sahra Kırmusaoğlu

Notice

Statements and opinions expressed in the chapters are these of the individual contributors and not necessarily those of the editors or publisher. No responsibility is accepted for the accuracy of information contained in the published chapters. The publisher assumes no responsibility for any damage or injury to persons or property arising out of the use of any materials, instructions, methods or ideas contained in the book.

First published in London, United Kingdom, 2018 by IntechOpen
IntechOpen is the global imprint of INTECHOPEN LIMITED, registered in England and Wales, registration number: 11086078, The Shard, 25th floor, 32 London Bridge Street
London, SE19SG – United Kingdom
Printed in Croatia

British Library Cataloguing-in-Publication Data
A catalogue record for this book is available from the British Library

Additional hard copies can be obtained from orders@intechopen.com

Disinfection, Edited by Sahra Kırmusaoğlu
p. cm.
Print ISBN 978-1-78984-474-0
Online ISBN 978-1-78984-475-7

We are IntechOpen,
the world's leading publisher of Open Access books
Built by scientists, for scientists

3,800+
Open access books available

116,000+
International authors and editors

120M+
Downloads

Our authors are among the

151
Countries delivered to

Top 1%
most cited scientists

12.2%
Contributors from top 500 universities

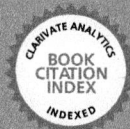

Interested in publishing with us?
Contact book.department@intechopen.com

Numbers displayed above are based on latest data collected.
For more information visit www.intechopen.com

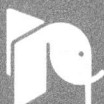

Meet the editor

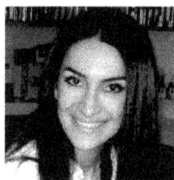

Dr. Kırmusaoğlu is an Assistant Professor of Microbiology at the Department of Molecular Biology and Genetics, T.C. Haliç University, where she had previously held an administrative position as vice head of the same department. She specialized in microbiology at Abant Izzet Baysal University (Biology Department), Turkey.

Her previous experience includes the position of laboratory manager at microbiology laboratories in several research and private hospitals. Throughout her career, she collaborated with academicians/researchers from AIBU, METU, and IU Cerrahpaşa Medical Faculty, and participated in various research projects. She also worked as a lecturer in the Medical Laboratory Techniques Program held at the Department of Medical Services and Techniques, T.C. Istanbul Kavram Vocational Training School before transitioning to T.C. Haliç University as an assistant professor. Dr. Kırmusaoğlu's research interests include pathogenic bacterial biofilms, antibiofilm and antimicrobial agents, and the effects and synergistic effects of new alternative agents such as chemical and natural bioactive compounds against pathogenic bacteria, such as antibiotic-resistant and biofilm-producing microorganisms. She is also interested in research on antibiofilm medical devices and food package design for preventing biofilm infections associated with indwelling devices that could lead to systemic infections, food-borne infections, and prolongation of foods' shelf life. She has published several international research articles, book chapters, and congress proceedings. More specifically, Dr. Kırmusaoğlu participated as an author in books entitled *Microbial Biofilms*: *Importance and Applications* and *Staphylococcus aureus* with her chapters "Staphylococcal Biofilms: Pathogenicity, Mechanism and Regulation of Biofilm Formation by Quorum Sensing System and Antibiotic Resistance Mechanisms of Biofilm Embedded Microorganisms" and "The Mechanism of Methicillin Resistance and the Influence of Methicillin Resistance on Biofilm Phenotype of Staphylococcus aureus". She is the editor of the book entitled *Bacterial Pathogenesis and Antibacterial Control* published by Intech. She is also the author and editor of the book entitled *Genel Biyoloji Laboratuvar Kılavuzu* (*General Biology Laboratory Manual*) published by Hipokrat Publisher. She has also been contributing to a book project entitled *Antimicrobials* as an editor, and has been contributing a chapter translation of the book entitled *Sherris Medical Microbiology* by Ryan et al. as one of the translation authors of *Sherris Medikal Mikrobiyoloji*, which will be a Turkish translated book.

Contents

Overview to Disinfection

Chapter 1

Introductory Chapter: Overview of Disinfection

Sahra Kırmusaoğlu

Additional information is available at the end of the chapter

http://dx.doi.org/10.5772/intechopen.81051

1. Introduction

1.1. Importance of disinfection

Disinfection is the method to destroy most microbial forms, especially vegetative pathogens rather than bacterial spores, by using physical and chemical procedures such as UV radiation, boiling, vapor. Each surgical process and medical applications need sterile procedures to avoid infection of tissue by surgical and medical equipment that are contaminated. During these processes, surgical and medical equipment can be contaminated by pathogens via contaminated surgical gloves. This leads to entrance of bacteria adhered on surgical and medical equipment or devices to sterile tissues of patient as a result of infection. Not only contaminated surgical and medical equipment are risk factors for infection but also contaminated common areas used by community such as toilets, public transport vehicles and door handles and contaminated air causing transmission of pathogens from person to person and contaminated kitchen equipment causing cross contamination between equipment and foods are risk factors for health-threatening infections. Inadequate disinfections of these equipment and air are risk factors for transmission of pathogens to patients. Hepatitis B, hepatitis C, Rota virus, *Staphylococcus aureus*, *Staphylococcus epidermidis*, *Escherichia coli* O157:H7, *Salmonella typhimurium*, *Shigella dysenteriae*, *Vibrio cholera*, and *Helicobacter pylori* are the most common examples of pathogens transmitted. Failure to apply disinfection applications has been leading to various outbreaks [1].

2. Guidelines for disinfection applications

There are many guidelines for choosing and using proper disinfection and sterilization methods by effective disinfectants in distinct areas, and application of disinfection and sterilization methods in many countries, such as Centers for Disease Control and Prevention (CDC), and the Society for Healthcare Epidemiology of America (SHEA). Guideline for Disinfection and Sterilization in Healthcare Facilities that searched and used articles published in American Journal of Infection Control, Infection Control and Hospital Epidemiology, and Journal of Hospital Infection that are the three common journals for controlling infection was written by Rutala and Weber (2008 and updated in February 15, 2017) and published by CDC [1].

3. Disinfectants

Contaminated biotic surfaces such as skin, contaminated abiotic surfaces such as medical devices, and kitchen equipment exposed to cross contamination must be disinfected to prevent pathogens. Alcohols, chlorine and chlorine compounds, quaternary ammonium compounds, phenolics, iodophors, formaldehyde, glutaraldehyde, *ortho*-phthalaldehyde, hydrogen peroxide, peracetic acid are examples of disinfectants used. Microbicide metals, ultraviolet radiation (UV), pasteurization were also used for disinfection of surfaces, as miscellaneous inactivating agents [1].

4. Efficacy of disinfection

Bactericidal effects of disinfectants vary against each microorganism. According to efficacy of disinfectant, appropriate disinfectant must be used against each microorganism. For example, a few types of disinfectants are not suitable for cold, due to inefficacy of disinfectant at lower temperatures of environment. This problem can be overcome by selecting appropriate disinfectant of which effect is high in cold conditions [2, 3].

Temperature and pH of the disinfection process, amount of microorganism, physical factors such as surface type, chemical factors such as chemical composition of surface or disinfectant, antibacterial resistance of microorganism, biofilm production of microorganism, dose of disinfection, and duration of exposure to disinfection are the factors affecting efficacy of disinfectant against pathogens [1].

Susceptibilities of biofilm-embedded bacteria (sessile cells) and spores to disinfectants are lesser than planktonic and vegetative cells. It is hard to destroy bacterial biofilms, bacterial spores, and resistant microorganisms that can stay alive. Bacterial spores and resistant microorganisms can resist disinfectants. Studies showed that the effect of some disinfectants such as chlorhexidine, propamidine, and quaternary ammonium compound cetrimide against methicillin-sensitive *Staphylococcus aureus* (MSSA) was greater than that of methicillin-resistant *Staphylococcus aureus* (MRSA) which is a life-threatening pathogen [4]. Researchers found that the susceptibility of gentamicin-resistant *Staphylococcus aureus* (*S. aureus*) isolates against propamidine, quaternary ammonium compounds, and ethidium bromide was lesser than gentamicin-susceptible *S. aureus* isolates [5]. Tennent et al. demonstrated that the susceptibility of staphylococci carrying *qac*A gene that encodes cytoplasmic membrane-associated protein which is a member of an efflux system was reduced against some disinfectants such as quaternary ammonium compounds [6].

In contrary to these studies, some other studies demonstrated that susceptibility of common antibiotic-resistant nosocomial isolates such as *Enterococcus, Pseudomonas aeruginosa, Klebsiella pneumoniae, E. coli, S. aureus*, and *Staphylococcus epidermidis* against disinfectants was the same as antibiotic-sensitive ones [7–10]. Other studies concluded that vancomycin-resistant *Enterococcus* (VRE) was eliminated by disinfectants [11].

Although biofilm-embedded bacteria are 10- to 1000-fold more resistant than planktonic ones [12], disinfectants such as chlorine and monochloramines eliminate biofilm-embedded bacteria [13–15].

Author details

Sahra Kırmusaoğlu

Address all correspondence to: kirmusaoglu_sahra@hotmail.com

Department of Molecular Biology and Genetics, Faculty of Arts and Science, T.C. Halic University, Istanbul, Turkey

References

[1] Rutala WA, Weber DJ. Guideline for Disinfection and Sterilization in Healthcare Facilities, Centers for Disease Control and Prevention. CDC; 2008. p. 161 (updated in Feburary 15, 2017) Available from: https://www.cdc.gov/infectioncontrol/guidelines/disinfection/

[2] Lelieveld HL, Holah J, Gabric D. Handbook of Hygiene Control in the Food Industry. Woodhead Publishing; 2016

[3] Lelieveld HL, Holah J, Napper D, editors. Hygiene in Food Processing: Principles and Practice. Elsevier; 2014

[4] Brumfitt W, Dixson S, Hamilton-Miller JM. Resistance to antiseptics in methicillin and gentamicin resistant *Staphylococcus aureus*. Lancet. 1985;**1**:1442-1443

[5] Townsend DE, Ashdown N, Greed LC, Grubb WB. Transposition of gentamicin resistance to staphylococcal plasmids encoding resistance to cationic agents. The Journal of Antimicrobial Chemotherapy. 1984;**14**:115-124

[6] Tennent JM, Lyon BR, Midgley M, Jones IG, Purewal AS, Skurray RA. Physical and biochemical characterization of the qacA gene encoding antiseptic and disinfectant resistance in *Staphylococcus aureus*. Journal of General Microbiology. 1989;**135**:1-10

[7] Rutala WA, Barbee SL, Aguiar NC, Sobsey MD, Weber DJ. Antimicrobial activity of home disinfectants and natural products against potential human pathogens. Infection Control and Hospital Epidemiology. 2000;**21**:33-38

[8] Rutala WA, Stiegel MM, Sarubbi FA, Weber DJ. Susceptibility of antibiotic-susceptible and antibiotic-resistant hospital bacteria to disinfectants. Infection Control and Hospital Epidemiology. 1997;**18**:417-421

[9] Anderson RL, Carr JH, Bond WW, Favero MS. Susceptibility of vancomycin-resistant enterococci to environmental disinfectants. Infection Control and Hospital Epidemiology. 1997;**18**:195-199

[10] Sakagami Y, Kajimura K. Bactericidal activities of disinfectants against vancomycin-resistant enterococci. The Journal of Hospital Infection. 2002;**50**:140-144

[11] Rutala WA, Weber DJ, Gergen MF. Studies on the disinfection of VRE-contaminated surfaces. Infection Control and Hospital Epidemiology. 2000;**21**:548

[12] Marion K, Freney J, James G, Bergeron E, Renaud FNR, Costerton JW. Using an efficient biofilm detaching agent: An essential step for the improvement of endoscope reprocessing protocols. Journal of Hospital Infection. 2006;**64**(2):136-142

[13] Donlan RM, Costerton JW. Biofilms: Survival mechanisms of clinically relevant mirocorganisms. Clinical Microbiology Reviews. 2002;**15**:167-193

[14] Vickery K, Pajkos A, Cossart Y. Removal of biofilm from endoscopes: Evaluation of detergent efficiency. American Journal of Infection Control. 2004;**32**:170-176

[15] Marion-Ferey K, Pasmore M, Stoodley P, Wilson S, Husson GP, Costerton JW. Biofilm removal from silicone tubing: An assessment of the efficacy of dialysis machine decontamination procedures using an *in vitro* model. The Journal of Hospital Infection. 2003;**53**:64-71

Disinfection of Water

Chapter 2

Disinfection of Water Used for Human and Animal Consumption

Tatiana Hrušková, Naďa Sasáková,
Gabriela Gregová, Ingrid Papajová and
Zuzana Bujdošová

Additional information is available at the end of the chapter

http://dx.doi.org/10.5772/intechopen.76430

Abstract

This chapter deals with disinfection of water used for human and animal consumption. Water is the most abundant chemical component of the Earth and is very extensively used by mankind. Anthropogenic pressure on the environment leads to decrease in water quality. The quality of water is determined using the most important range of parameters (physical, chemical, and microbiological). This chapter discusses major pollutants of water, protection of water sources, micro-organisms causing the main waterborne diseases and methods of treatment, and disinfection of water. Different methods are used to disinfect drinking water. One of the most frequently used methods is disinfection with active chlorine, which is the only method providing continuous protection against microbial regrowth. However, this method has also some disadvantages (e.g., formation of trihalomethane and haloacetic acid precursors) linked to increased risk of cancer. It is important to remember that none of the products used to disinfect water is capable of ensuring complete safety of treated water if the water comes from unsuitable sources.

Keywords: disinfection, chlorination, drinking water safety, farm animal watering, microbiological examination, physico-chemical examination

1. Introduction

Water is essential for the existence of life. It should be available to all at adequate quantity and quality. Access to safe drinking water is the basic requirement for ensuring good health of animals and humans, so every effort should be made to achieve this goal [1]. The safety of drinking water is assessed on the basis of national standards or international guidelines. The WHO Guidelines for Drinking Water Quality form an authoritative basis for the setting of national regulations and standards for water safety in support of public health. In Slovakia, regulation of the government of the SR Act No. 368/2007 Coll. [2], which amends and supplements the Act No. 322/2003 Coll. [3], on protection of farm animals, specifies that all sources of water used for watering of animals must comply with the requirements on water intended for human consumption. The requirements on the quality of water used for human consumption are determined by the regulation of the government of the SR No. 496/2010 Coll. [4], which complies with the criteria set by European Communities regulations and WHO guidelines. This regulation specifies also methods for the control of quality of water used for human consumption.

Water sources can be contaminated by numerous man-made pollutants, classified into two categories of sources, point and diffuse. Industrial premises, towns, agricultural installations including animal farms and landfills—point sources—can be more easily identified and controlled. Diffuse sources, such as run-off from agricultural land and hard surfaces (roads and acid rains), are less obvious and more difficult to control. Such sources are responsible for considerable variations in the contaminant load over time [5].

Source protection zones (SPZs) form a key part of the approach to controlling the risk to groundwater supplies from potentially polluting activities and accidental releases of pollutants. The procedure for land-surface zoning related to the protection of groundwater against both point and diffuse pollution is hydrogeologically based but not so complex as to be unworkable in practice. The SPZ approach is primarily a policy tool used to control activities close to water supplies intended for human consumption. For source protection, three zones have typically been defined:

1. Inner protection zone is defined as the 50-day travel time from any point below the water table to the source. The minimum radius of this zone is 50 m.

2. Outer protection zone is defined by a 400-day travel time from a point below the water table.

3. Source catchment protection zone is defined as the area around a source within which all groundwater recharge is presumed to be discharged at the source.

In the case of diffuse pollution, it will also be necessary to consider the nature of the soil cover in the area where the polluting activity occurs [6, 7].

Many agents of infectious diseases of animals and humans are waterborne. The greatest risk of their transfer is associated with ingestion of water that is contaminated with human or animal faeces that may become a source of pathogenic bacteria, viruses, and parasites (protozoa, eggs of parasites). They may survive in water for different periods and cause diseases in many people throughout the world. Monitoring of safety of water sources involves physical, chemical, microbiological, biological, and radiological parameters. The most frequently determined parameters indicate pollution caused by sewage, animal excrements, storage of waste, animal manure, and artificial fertilisers [8, 9]. With regard to protection of water, one should also mention the Directive 2010/75/EU [10] on integrated prevention of pollution and control that applies to industrial and agricultural installations with large pollution potential and helps to eliminate pollution of water sources. However, there are many smaller sources, particularly the non-point ones that do not fall under this directive.

The safety of drinking water with regard to harmful micro-organisms has traditionally been determined by monitoring the counts of bacteria, which indicate faecal contamination. This monitoring is done at entry to the supply system and at certain fixed and randomly located points within the distribution system. Much effort has been made to find ideal indicator micro-organisms, but, at present, no single micro-organism meets satisfactorily all the desired criteria. When using disinfection technologies based on active chlorine, the only reliable indicator of chlorination performance for real-time control of bacteria and viruses is the existence of a target chlorine residual concentration after a specified contact time [7].

The heterotrophic plate count that includes all micro-organisms in water capable of growing on or in a nutrient-rich solid agar is determined to indicate the overall quality of water sources. At incubation for 24 hours at a temperature of 37°C (bacteria cultivated at 37°C, BC37), the counts of bacteria of animal origin are obtained, while at 22°C and cultivation for 72 hours (bacteria cultivated at 22°C, BC22), one can enumerate bacteria that are derived principally from environmental sources. Substantial increase of BC22 and particularly of BC37 above, normal values may be cause for concern. Faecal enterococci as an evidence of faecal contamination are capable of persisting longer in the environment in comparison with thermotolerant or total coliforms. They exhibit high resistance to drying. Faecal enterococci are cultivated in or on sodium azide containing medium, at incubation temperature ranging from 37 to 44°C [11].

According to WHO [12], *Escherichia coli* are the only true indicator of faecal contamination. These bacteria are exclusively of intestinal origin and are found in human and animal faeces. They are indicators of mostly fresh faecal contamination, and their presence suggests inadequate protection of the specific water source, deficient treatment of water, and need for improving its safety.

Leclerc et al. [13] clarified the diversified roles that coliforms have in the environment and the real meanings of the tests on total coliforms and faecal coliforms. He concluded that: (1) in the enterobacteria, *E. coli* are the only true and reliable indicator of faecal pollution in environmental waters; (2) the traditional total coliform test should be abandoned because it can detect bacteria that have no connection with faecal pollution; (3) the detection of faecal coliforms must be carried out at 44.5°C, and positive results confirmed by identification to species levels in order to exclude false positives such as *Klebsiella pneumoniae*.

The intestinal enterococci group has been used as an index of faecal pollution. In human faeces, the numbers of intestinal enterococci are generally about an order of magnitude lower than those of *E. coli*. However, caution should be taken with interpreting the results obtained by the enterococci procedure in water analysis. Enterococci and other group D-streptococci are present in many foods, especially those of animal origin [14].

Managing microbial risks in water supply relies primarily on identifying catchment risk and, as far as possible, applying control measures to mitigate it—treatment and disinfection systems designed to deal effectively with expected microbial loads, raw water quality, preventing microbial contamination in distribution system and at consumers. This is consistent with the Drinking Water Safety Plan (DWSP) approach for water supply risk, which is a risk-based approach to managing water quality that is designed to ensure delivery of safe drinking water in terms of both quality and quantity. Then, effectiveness of controls and barriers has to be validated and action plan to reduce risks to an acceptable level identified [7].

The physico-chemical properties of water, particularly pH, temperature, the presence of organic matter (chemical oxygen demand, COD), low level of dissolved oxygen (DO), electric conductivity (EC), turbidity, content of ammonium ion, presence of heavy metals, and others, affect the quality of drinking water, and some of them have direct effect on the health of consumers [15]. In addition, these parameters can affect the survival of potential disease agents, the effectiveness of the performed disinfection [16].

Although the groundwater is filtered when passing through the soil, it is often susceptible to microbial contamination and must be checked periodically and disinfected if necessary. A major groundwater pathogen occurrence study supported by the American Water Works Association (AWWA) Research Foundation and the U.S. Environmental Protection Agency (EPA), involving testing for total coliform bacteria, E. coli, coliphage, and human viruses, indicated positivity for one or more indicators of faecal contamination that in 60% of vulnerable wells and about 50% of wells initially considered not vulnerable.

1.1. Disinfection of drinking water

The current drinking water regulations specify parametric values for various chemicals in drinking water, and compliance with the limits for microbiological parameters is of primary concern in the protection of human health. Different disinfectant technologies can be used to eliminate the risks consequent to the presence of organic and inorganic impurities in source waters and to meet the pathogen inactivation demands, as a part of a treatment process and/or subsequent disinfection processes.

The control of residual organic or inorganic compounds in water before disinfection limits disinfection by-products in water supplied to consumers. The maintenance of a disinfectant residual within the distribution system that is not ensured by all disinfection technologies is an important factor that prevents the regrowth of microorganisms in water.

The following key factors influence the selection of a disinfection system: the effectiveness of the disinfectant in destroying pathogens of concern; the quality of the water to be disinfected; the formation of undesirable by-products as a result of disinfection; the ability to easily verify the operation of the chosen disinfection system; the ease of handling and health and safety implications of a disinfectant; the preceding treatment processes; and the overall cost [7].

Chlorination is a chemical disinfection based on the application of various substances with different concentration of active chlorine ranging from gaseous chlorine, through sodium or calcium hypochlorite and chloramines, up to chlorine dioxide. Chlorine-based compounds are the only major disinfectants ensuring residual levels of the disinfectant agent capable of providing continuous protection against microbial regrowth [17].

When chlorination is performed with gas chlorine, the active forms of chlorine in water are a hydrolysis product, hypochlorous acid. At pH values below 6, the chlorine exists almost exclusively as hypochlorous acid, and at pH values above 9, it exists as hypochlorite. Since hypochlorous acid is a more potent disinfectant, chlorination under slightly acidic conditions is recommended [18].

The dose of chlorine is affected by the quality of the treated water and the form of the chlorine preparation used for disinfection. The above factors affect the residual active chlorine levels present in water supplied to the consumer. Active chlorine preparations have been considered the most suitable way of disinfection of on-farm groundwater (wells) for numerous reasons. Such disinfection is cost effective, reliable, relatively simple, measurable and provides a protective residual level of active chlorine [17, 19].

Different techniques of chlorination have been developed. Breakpoint chlorination uses active chlorine dose sufficient to rapidly oxidise all the ammonia nitrogen present in the water and to leave free residual chlorine capable of protecting the water against reinfection from the point of disinfection always up to the consumer. Superchlorination/dechlorination is based on the addition of a large dose of chlorine ensuring rapid disinfection by-products of relevant chemical reaction, followed by reduction in the excess of free chlorine residual, which must be removed to prevent taste problems and reduce corrosion of pipelines. The latter method is used mainly in case of variable bacterial load or inadequate detention time in the tank. Marginal chlorination is used for disinfection of high quality water supplies. It involves simple dosing of chlorine to produce a desired level of free residual chlorine. The chlorine demand of water from these sources is very low, and the breakpoint might not even occur [1].

The original WHO recommendations for the use of chlorine as a disinfectant stipulated a minimum free chlorine concentration of 0.5 mg/L after 30 min contact time at a pH of less than 8 provided that the turbidity is less than 1 nephelometric turbidity unit (NTU). A site specific approach may need to take into account: the levels of contamination with pathogens expected, and any specific pathogens of concern for the site (catchment risk); the extent and performance of treatment prior to final disinfection; the design of the contact tank, in relation to short-circuiting; and expected variations in temperature and pH [7].

The by-products (BPs) of chlorine disinfectants can affect the health of consumers of the disinfected water or induce in them various responses. Their extent depends on numerous factors such as the period of action, concentration, and frequency of exposure [20].

Chlorine dioxide is a more powerful disinfectant than chlorine and does not form trihalomethanes (THMs) by reaction with humic substances. However, its generation is also associated with some BPs, such as chlorites and chlorates [21]. One of the most undesirable BPs in generators is the toxic chlorate ion [18]. It cannot be stored in compressed form in tanks because it is explosive under pressure and must be generated on site and thus is likely to be substantially more expensive than chlorine.

Chloramination of water is based on the formation of monochloramine, which is formed when ammonia and chlorine are dosed, and react, under well-controlled conditions. It is essential to control the process to prevent the formation of strong tastes and by-products. The disinfection capability of monochloramine is poor when compared with chlorine. The key advantage of monochloramine is that it does not form THMs but still provides a disinfectant residual [7].

Chloramine-T is an organic N-chloramine. Chloramine-T is a slow-release chlorinating agent, and it is an exception to the organic chloramines because of its considerable value as a disinfectant and a sanitiser. The hydrolysis mechanism involves the production of aqueous free chlorine ($HClO$, ClO^-). Organic chloramines in general are thought to be considerably less toxic to aquatic life than the inorganic chloramines, such as mono-, di-, and trichloramine. Inorganic chloramines usually exist as monochloramine in aqueous solutions [22]. The detailed hydrolysis mechanism of chloramine-T varies with pH and is quite complex. In aqueous solutions of chloramine-T, caused by dissociation, hydrolysis, and disproportionation processes, seven different kinds of molecules emerge (HClO, ClO$^-$, R—NCl—, R—NHCl, R—NCl$_2$, R—NH$_2$, and R—NH—[R=CH$_3$—C$_6$H$_4$—SO$_2$]) [23]. The use of chloramine-T solutions for disinfection of water includes its use in aquaculture. Tests performed on brook trout by Cipriano et al. [24] substantiated the therapeutic value of single treatment with chloramine-T (15 mg/L) against *Aeromonas salmonicida*, which was more successful than that treatment with formalin or salt.

Schmidt et al. [22] presented detailed environmental assessment of the effects of chloramine-T use in and discharge by freshwater aquaculture. Intensive aquaculture facilities discharge into streams, rivers, and lakes. Both before and after discharge, chloramine-T can remain unchanged, release its chlorine as aqueous free chlorine, or donate its chlorine directly to produce ammonia chloramines or other chlorinated organic-N or non-N compounds. Since chloramine-T is used as an antiseptic and a surface sanitising agent, toxicity to bacteria is to be expected at some concentration level. Chloramine-T was an effective microbicide against *Pseudomonas aeruginosa* at 300 mg/L (reduced colony forming units by 10^5) and at 5000 mg/L against *Vibrio cholerae* [25].

Ozone is more powerful disinfectant when compared with either chlorine or chlorine dioxide. It is the only chemical that can ensure effective inactivation of either Giardia or Cryptosporidium. It also destructs organic micropollutants (pesticides, odour compounds). However, its residual is insufficiently low lasting for distribution.

The non-chemical disinfection system involves ultraviolet (UV) radiation. It is necessary to ensure suitable intensity and duration of UV radiation to give a UV "dose," which will depend on the application. Dose of 40 mJ/cm^2 is commonly used for UV disinfection systems as it is capable of inactivating a broad spectrum of waterborne pathogens. It is effective for protozoa, bacteria, and most viruses but less effective for viruses than chlorine [7].

The main drawback of disinfection with gaseous chlorine and active chlorine releasing preparations is that chlorine can react with natural organic matter (NOM) present in water to generate various types of disinfection BPs, such as trihalomethane and haloacetic acid. The BPs are associated with increased incidence of the risk of cancer in areas served with chlorinated water [26, 27]. Zhao et al. [28] mentioned chloro- and bromobenzochinones as additional by-products of chlorination.

The presence of NOM in water and their chemical and physical characteristics can be investigated by excitation emission matrix (EEM) fluorescence spectroscopy that serves as a powerful tool [27].

As the effectiveness of chlorination can be affected by NOM, it is important to obtain adequate information about this parameter. As the content of NOM in water from natural sources may vary considerably, the optimum dose of chlorine disinfectants necessary for complying with the respective legislative requirements on active chlorine residuals should be determined, for example, by experimental chlorination [29].

With regard to the negative effects of gaseous chlorine and stricter legislation, new methods and technological procedures were searched for to find a way of ensuring hygiene safety of drinking water. Of the physical methods, Jirotkova et al. [30] proposed the use of electrolytic methods, and Hussain et al. [31] presented the combination of adsorption and electrochemical disinfection. Recently, UV technologies with online fluorescence detection were employed for disinfection of secondary water sources [32], for example, the combination of mechanical filtration and disinfection by solar radiation [33], or combined action of UV radiation and chlorine [34]. With these new approaches, one could achieve reduction in the level of undesirable BPs and elimination of negative effects on physical properties of water, resembling that after disinfection with ozone [35]. However, the majority of them do not ensure the residual disinfection power.

The aim of this study was to monitor the quality and safety of three groundwater sources located in the eastern Slovakia and to determine experimentally the optimum dose of chloramine-T (commercial preparation) needed for their adequate disinfection that could ensure hygiene safety of water in terms of devitalisation of potential pathogens and observation of the relevant limit for residual active chlorine (0.3 mg/L) in drinking water [36].

2. Materials and methods

The study involved monitoring of three groundwater sources supplying water to three farms, two cattle farms, and one farm keeping both cattle and sheep, located in a hilly area in the Prešov region (eastern Slovakia), about 4 km apart. The samples of groundwater from these wells were collected from January to May, in intervals specified below. The quality of water in the investigated sources and its potential to form disinfectant BPs was assessed on the basis of microbiological, physico-chemical, and fluorescence analyses. After obtaining unfavourable bacteriological results during preliminary sampling in January and February, experimental chlorination of water was carried out for each source. Subsequently, the effectiveness of such dose was then checked under field conditions.

The experimental chlorination was conducted using a chloramine-T (sodium tosylchloramid; sodium salt of N-chloro-4-methylbenzene-1-sulfonamide) as disinfectant. It involves the determination of optimum dose of chloramine T and intervals between application of this disinfectant necessary to prevent transmission of waterborne diseases and ensure such level of residual chlorine, so that the water can be used for watering of animals (complying with the national limit for residual active chlorine 0.3 mg/L) and for other related processes [37, 38].

2.1. Description of the monitored water sources

Source 1: It was located on a farm in eastern Slovakia at a distance of approximately 13 km from the town Prešov. The farm focused on fattening and rearing of cattle and included milk-producing dairy cows and a calf rearing section. The farm was well-known abroad because of fattening of bulls [39]. Five groundwater sources with a capacity of about 8000 L/d and depth in the range of 6–11 m were situated in close proximity of this farm. Water from these wells was brought to a storage tank of capacity about 40,000 L/d, from which the water was supplied to animals and used for other related operations. Water samples were collected from the common storage tank.

Source 2: It was located on a farm situated 15 km northeast of Prešov. Sheep of Tsigai breed and Slovak-spotted cattle were kept on this farm. The source was a 23-m deep well. Water from this well was collected in a storage reservoir located up on a hill above the farm, of capacity 150,000 L/d. Water samples were collected from the storage reservoir.

Source 3: A well of depth of 20 m and a reservoir of capacity of about 90,000 L/d were located on a farm 12.5 km away from Prešov. On this farm, young cattle and dairy cows were kept. The water samples for examination were collected from a tap in a cow house.

2.2. Microbiological examination

Determination of counts of relevant bacteria complied with the regulation of the government of the SR 496/2010 Coll. We determined colony forming units (CFUs) of bacteria cultivated at 22°C (BC22) and 37°C (BC37) (heterotrophic count) according to STN EN ISO 6222 [7], coliform bacteria (CB) and *E. coli* according to STN EN ISO 9308–1 [40], and faecal enterococci (FE) according to STN EN ISO 7899–2 [41]. A pour-plate method was used to determine counts of BC22 and BC37 in nutrient agar medium after aerobic incubation. The number of colony forming units (CFUs) per mL of sample was determined. According to the regulation of the government of the SR 496/2010 Coll. [4], the limit value is 200 CFU/mL for BC22 and 20 CFU/mL for BC37.

Coliform bacteria (CB) and *E. coli* were cultivated on Endo agar (HiMedia, India) for 24 hours at 37 and 43°C, respectively, and the characteristic colonies were counted. In the absence of colonies, the incubation was prolonged for additional 24 hours. According to respective regulation, lactose fermentation test was performed for the confirmation of coliform bacteria. According to WHO (2008) [1], neither *E. coli* nor thermotolerant coliform bacteria can be detected in any 100-mL sample. The same applies to total coliform bacteria that must not be detected in any 100-mL sample (WHO, 1996, STN EN ISO 9308-1:90) [11, 40].

Determination of faecal enterococci (FE) consisted of filtering 100 or 10 mL of water sample (for water intended for mass consumption or individual consumption, respectively) through a membrane filter (filter size 0.45 μm). The filter was then placed onto a solid selective medium containing sodium azide (to suppress growth of Gram-negative bacteria) and colourless 2,3,5-trifenyltetrazolium chloride, which is reduced by intestinal enterococci to red formazan. The regulation stipulates that faecal enterococci must not be detected in any 100 mL sample of water [42].

2.3. Experimental chlorination of water

The preliminary bacteriological examination of water from all three sources showed the need to carry out experimental chlorination of water. This allowed us to determine appropriate doses of chloramine-T necessary for disinfection of water in the investigated sources.

Procedure—Horakova et al. [29]: We used 0.1% solution of chloramine-T for experimental chlorination (active ingredient Tosylchloramide sodium, 81% active chlorine, manufactured by Bochemie—http://www.bochemie.cz/en-US/contact) [43]. The dosage recommended by the manufacturer is 10 g per 1000 L of water (this presumes maximum pollution of water). After measuring equal volumes of water into a series of bottles, we added to them increasing doses of 0.1% solution of chloramine-T, allowed it to act for the prescribed time (30 min) and determined content of residual free chlorine in each bottle. The optimum dose of chloramine-T (g/L) for each source was determined by recalculation on the basis of the volume of 0.1% chloramine-T added to the bottle with the residual free chlorine within the range stipulated by the legislation (0.05–0.3 mg/L).

The doses of chloramine-T determined by experimental chlorination and dissolved in a sufficient volume of water before added to each source were used to disinfect water in the investigated sources three times in regular intervals during the first half of 2015. On the 5th day after disinfection, we carried out bacteriological examination of water. On the basis of results, the chloramine-T dose originally determined by experimental chlorination (100 g) for Source 1—100 were doubled after heavy rain in April to 200 g. The dose for Source 2 was 360 g for reservoir with a capacity of about 150,000 L/d and 180 g (90,000 L/d) for Source 3.

2.4. Physico-chemical examination of water

The water was examined on site for sensorial properties (colour, odour, turbidity) and checked again after transported to a laboratory. No changes were detected, and the results met the requirements set by legislation for drinking water. The temperature of samples was measured at sampling and ranged between 7 and 10.5°C. Water was sampled and examined from January to May 2015.

The pH was determined according to STN ISO 10523 by means of a pH-meter HACH and a WATERPROF pH Tester 30. Conductivity was determined by a conductometer WTW InoLab Cond 720 (Germany).

Quantitative determination of nitrates was carried out with ion-selective nitrate electrode WTW (InoLab pH/ION 735P, Germany), and chlorides and active chlorine were determined by titration (STN ISO 9297 [44] and EN ISO 7393-3 [45], respectively) and Ca^{2+} and Mg^{2+} by titration method according to Horakova et al. [29]. Dissolved oxygen was determined electrochemically using an oxygen probe LDO HQ Series Portable Meters, supplied by HACH (STN EN ISO 5814:2013 [46], ion selective method), and for determination of chemical oxygen demand, the samples were oxidisied with $KMnO_4$ using the procedure specified in STN EN ISO 8467 [47].

In parallel with collection of samples for microbiological and physico-chemical analysis, samples of water from all three water sources were taken for FEEM spectroscopy and examined by a luminescence spectrophotometer Perkin Elmer LS 55 (USA) at the following settings: excitation wavelength in the range 250–450 nm with a gradual increment increase (10 nm), range λ = 250–600 nm (excitation/emission slit: 5/10 nm, quartz cuvette of width 1 cm, scanning rate of emission monochromator: 20 nm/s). Excitation-emission matrices (EEMs) were obtained using a FIW Inlab programme [48].

3. Results and discussion

Water problems face virtually every nation in the world. Major water supply problems are related to shortages, overexploitation of supplies, flooding and insufficient protection of water sources, either surface or ground, against contamination with human and animal wastes, and other human activities. Good quality of water intended for human consumption and watering of animals is essential for its safety and prevention of disease transfer.

Surface water serves as a recipient not only for rain water from relevant catchment areas but also of wastewater (treated and untreated) and waters penetrated by infiltration from landfills. Because removal of some pollutants is very difficult and expensive, pollution of surface water that is used for drinking after appropriate treatment must be prevented. This is achieved by zones of protection, the size of which depends on particular situation [18].

The primary pollution of groundwater can be caused by substances naturally occurring in groundwater and the mineral environment or by all types of wastewater, industry, agriculture, transportation, and exploitation of minerals. Therefore, groundwater sources also require protection, regular monitoring, and some treatment—the process of converting raw water from subsurface source into a potable form, suitable for drinking and other domestic uses. The method used for the treatment of groundwater will depend on the contaminants involved [49]. Although scientists look for new methods of disinfection or combine several technologies in order to reduce some harmful by-products associated with some ways of disinfection [50], processes based on active chlorine releasing substances are still most frequently used owing to their effectiveness, relatively low cost and residual disinfection power.

3.1. Results of microbiological examination of disinfected groundwater

Because we monitored water that should meet the limits for drinking water, we compared our results with those set by the relevant legislation Act 496/2010 Coll. [1, 4, 11, 40].

3.1.1. Source 1

In the period from January to May 2015, this source was disinfected five times, and on 5th day post each chlorination, the bacteriological quality of water was checked. The results are presented in **Table 1**.

The first chlorination was performed using 20 g of chloramine-T dose for one well, based on previous experimental chlorination. Because bacteriological results obtained 5 days after

Parameter	CB (CFU)	E. coli (CFU)	BC 37 (CFU)	BC 22 (CFU)	FE (CFU)	Cl_2 (mg/L)
Before disinfection						
Mean value	160	1	18	23	1	0
5 days after disinfection by chloramine-T						
1 sample (20 g)	130	0	42	2	5	0
2 sample (40 g)	15	0	12	15	0	0
3 sample (40 g)	0	0	0	2	2	0
4 sample (40 g)	21	0	6	8	0	0
5 sample (40 g)	0	0	0	3	1	0.05
Limit (CFU)	0[a]	0[a]	20[b]	200[b]	0[a]	0.05–0.3

[a]CFU in 100 ml.
[b]CFU in 1 ml.
CB: coliform bacteria; BC 37 or BC 22: bacteria cultivated at 37 or 22°C; FE: faecal enterococci; Cl_2: free chlorine; CFU: colony forming unit.

Table 1. Results of microbiological examination and the level of free chlorine for Source 1 before and after disinfection with chloramine-T.

the first chlorination indicated that the dose cannot ensure effective disinfection, this dose was doubled in subsequent months to 40 g of chloramine-T per well. After the 4th chlorination, we observed that at the beginning of May no residual chlorine was present in water, and total coliform bacteria were detected in the relevant sample. Their presence suggested that a source of pollution may exist in the vicinity of one or more wells and that this source should be identified and eliminated in order to ensure safety of water. After the fifth chlorination at the end of May, before which there was a period without precipitations, the 40 g dose of chloramine-T appeared sufficient again. The wells that supplied water to the reservoir were not very deep (6–11 m), so in the period of intensive precipitations, they were more susceptible to contamination with various groups of bacteria including those of faecal origin, which could reach through run-off the relevant aquifer, as the wells were situated in an agricultural area. In such periods, we recommend more frequent disinfection of water with the 40 g dose.

Bonton et al. [51] observed that bacteriological pollution of groundwater in an agricultural area varied in space and time, and its contamination was higher during summer. Contamination exceeding the drinking water standard for treated water was determined in only 2% of the raw water samples. Total coliforms appeared to be a good precursor of *E. coli* or enterococci contamination.

Cho et al. [52] observed that heavy rainfall supports the transport of pathogenic bacteria. If these bacteria are introduced into groundwater, they can survive in a viable state but may or may not be culturable.

The studies of groundwater pollution focus usually on two to three indicator bacteria (e.g., total coliforms, faecal coliforms, and faecal enterococci) that were used to evaluate water quality. Because the combination of different kinds of pollution indicator bacteria provides better picture about faecal contamination in a given environment, we also used such approach in our study and determined heterotrophic counts besides indicator bacteria.

3.1.2. Source 2

After the experimental chlorination, Source 2 was disinfected with a dose of 180 g chloramine-T, which, however, appeared insufficient at checking on day 5 post disinfection as total coliforms and faecal coliforms were detected in the sample. This again required to increase the dose of chloramine-T to 360 g (**Table 2**). This increased dose was used in all four subsequent chlorinations and appeared effective up to May. After using 360 g dose, increased coliform counts were detected in this source at the beginning of May after intensive precipitations. Although the groundwater source has a depth of 23 m, it is located again in agricultural area where it can also run-off from the farm supplied from this source. Similar to the previous farm, change in intervals between disinfection is recommended in dependence on weather in order to ensure bacteriological safety of water.

3.1.3. Source 3

On the basis of experimental chlorination of water from Source 3, 180 g of chloramine-T was proposed as the optimum single dose. This amount was sufficient, and neither *E. coli* nor enterococci were detected after disinfection. The increased counts of coliform bacteria in the samples

Parameter	CB (CFU)	E. coli (CFU)	BC 37 (CFU)	BC 22 (CFU)	FE (CFU)	Cl_2 (mg/L)
Before disinfection						
Mean value	150	0	35	88	20	0
5 days after disinfection by chloramine-T						
1 sample (180 g)	55	0	195	192	2	0
2 sample (360 g)	1	0	32	125	0	0
3 sample (360 g)	1	0	15	30	0	0.05
4 sample (360 g)	8	0	85	136	0	0
5 sample (360 g)	0	0	0	2	0	0.15
Limit (CFU)	0[a]	0[a]	20[b]	200[b]	0[a]	0.05–0.3

[a]CFU in 100 ml.
[b]CFU in 1 ml.
CB: coliform bacteria; BC 37 or BC 22: bacteria cultivated at 37 or 22°C'; FE: faecal enterococci; Cl_2: free chlorine; CFU: colony forming unit.

Table 2. Results of microbiological examination and the level of free chlorine for Source 2 before and after disinfection with chloramine-T.

after fourth chlorination together with the detection of 1 CFU of *E. coli* and the absence of residual free chlorine could be ascribed to heavy rain, so more frequent disinfection is recommended in such period (**Table 3**).

Parameter	CB (CFU)	E. coli (CFU)	BC 37 (CFU)	BC 22 (CFU)	FE (CFU)	Cl_2 (mg/l)
Before disinfection						
Mean value	10	0	2	11	0	0
5 days after disinfection by chloramine-T						
1 sample (180 g)	1	0	3	8	0	0
2 sample (180 g)	3	1	0	19	1	0.05
3 sample (180 g)	2	0	0	12	0	0.05
4 sample (180 g)	9	1	13	38	0	0
5 sample (180 g)	0	0	1	2	0	0.05
Limit (CFU)	0[a]	0[a]	20[b]	200[b]	0[a]	0.05–0.3

[a]CFU in 100 ml.
[b]CFU in 1 ml.
CB: coliform bacteria; BC 37 or BC 22: bacteria cultivated at 37 or 22°C; FE: faecal enterococci; Cl_2: free chlorine; CFU: colony forming unit.

Table 3. Results of microbiological examination and the level of free chlorine for Source 3 before and after disinfection with chloramine-T.

Our results indicated better quality of water in this source in comparison with Sources 1 and 2. The depth of this source was considerable, and soil should ensure sufficient filtration of water. However, potential infiltration of pollutants is affected by many factors, such as the aquifer itself, immediate environment of well, geological conditions, existence of potential sources of pollution, and others.

3.2. Results of physico-chemical examination

Physico-chemical examination of water is important for assessment of its acceptability and potential health risks. Some chemical parameters indicate the risk of faecal or environmental contamination of water sources and may help to identify the sources of such contamination and take preventive measures.

Active chlorine added to water reacts to form hypochlorous acid and hypochlorite ion that are referred to as "free" or "available" chlorine. Their relative amounts vary with pH, when the pH rises above 8, the free chlorine loses most of its disinfectant power [53].

The presence of $N-NH_4^+$ in groundwaters is one of the most important indicators of fresh faecal pollution of water sources as a product of microbiological decomposition of organic matter and unused nutrients in the animal excrements. Although ammonium ions are retained by the cation exchange complex in the soil, Fridrich et al. [8] and Bartel-Hunt et al. [54] detected increased levels of ammonium nitrogen in shallow groundwater of the wells downstream from the pig housings and slurry lagoons. Natural levels of $N-NH_4^+$ in groundwater and surface water are usually below 0.2 mg/L, and anaerobic groundwaters may contain up to 3 mg/L [1].

Nitrates found in water as a final product of oxidation of $N-NH_4^+$ may also serve as indicators of older pollution. Due to various activities, such as excess application of inorganic nitrogenous fertilisers and animal manures, wastewater disposal, or leaking septic tanks, nitrates can reach both surface water and groundwater. While the concentration of nitrates in surface water can change rapidly as a result of run-off from the surface, application of fertilisers, uptake by phytoplankton, and action of denitrification bacteria, their concentrations in groundwater generally exhibit relatively slow changes. Although the most important sources of human exposure to nitrates and nitrites are vegetables and meat in the diet, under some circumstances, drinking water can significantly contribute to nitrate and, occasionally, nitrite intake [55]. Exposure of bottle-fed infants to nitrates and nitrites through drinking water can result in serious consequences.

In the majority of countries, the contribution of surface waters to nitrate levels in drinking water does not exceed 10 mg/L. However, nitrate levels in groundwater are often higher, exceeding the acceptable limit for adults (50 mg/L), particularly in agricultural areas. Nitrite levels are usually lower, rarely exceeding a few milligrammes per litre. Bonton et al. [51] monitored quality of groundwater and its variations in an agricultural area and reported considerable spatial and temporal variations in nitrate concentration from 6 to 125 mg/L.

Drinking water contains chlorides that originate from natural sources, sewage and industrial effluents, urban run-off containing de-icing salt, and saline intrusion. Urine of animals and humans contains relatively high levels of chlorides; therefore, values above 250 mg/L indicate risk of pollution of water with faeces [42].

The mineral content of natural and treated waters varies in considerable range. It could be important for individuals who are marginal for calcium and magnesium intake that drinking water may contribute to calcium and magnesium in the diet. Although epidemiological studies provided some information about a protective effect of magnesium or hardness on cardiovascular mortality, the evidence is being debated and does not prove causality. Further studies are being conducted in this respect. Because we lack sufficient data to suggest either minimum or maximum concentrations of minerals at this time, no guideline values for calcium and magnesium (hardness) are proposed [12].

Source 1: In water from Source 1, the pH was in the range of 6.9–7.4, which corresponded with the requirements on drinking water. Saturation with oxygen ranged from 55.4 to 80.9%. Saturation below the recommended level was determined in May (45.4% vs. recommended min. 50%), which could be related to intensive precipitations in the first half of this month. The contamination caused by increased run-off could result in processes with increased demand on oxygen.

Conductivity was in the range of 94.9–100.3 mS/m and was lower than the limit for this parameter (125 mS/m). Chemical oxygen demand ranged from 0.9 to 1.3 mg/L (limit 3.0 mg/L). Negative results were obtained for ammonium ions and nitrites. Nitrate levels ranged from 5.0 to 24 mg/L (limit 50 mg/L) and chlorides from 18.0 to 24.8 mg/L (limit 250 mg/L). Determination of calcium and magnesium showed that the recommended maximum concentration of these two elements (5 mmol/L) was exceeded at all samplings (5.18–5.78 mmol/L).

Contrary to the positive results for bacterial indicators, the physico-chemical examination of groundwater from Source 1 failed to indicate increased faecal contamination, even in the period of heavy precipitation.

Source 2: Determination of pH showed that all samples complied with the recommendations for drinking water. Level of dissolved oxygen (DO) in drinking water serves as an indication of its pollution and potability. Depletion of DO in water supplies can result in microbial reduction in nitrate to nitrite and sulphate to sulphide [1]. Saturation of water in this source was in the range of 81.9–95.6%, and thus well above the minimum limit, indicating good quality of water.

Electrical conductivity (EC) is a measure to the capacity of water to conduct electrical current, and it is directly related to the concentration of salts dissolved in water and therefore to the total dissolved solids (TDSs) principally calcium, magnesium, potassium, sodium, bicarbonates, chlorides, and sulphates and some small amounts of organic matter that are dissolved in water. The EC of the groundwater is a general indicator of manure pit leakage [56]. Conductivity of water in Source 2 ranged from 76.0 to 83.1 mS/m and complied with the standard (125 mS/m). Oxidisability (chemical oxygen demand $-COD_{Mn}$) ranged from 1.2 to 1.24 mg/L, i.e., well below the maximum limit (3.0 mg/L). The level of nitrates was in the range of 6–18 mg/L, i.e., well below the 50 mg/L limit. With regard to the level of calcium and magnesium, water from this reservoir was within the recommended range (1.1–5.0 mmol/L) as it ranged from 3.8 to 3.9 mmol/L.

Overall, similar to Source 1, the results of physico-chemical examination of water from Source 2 did not indicate significant pollution with faeces.

Source 3: pH values determined in all samples were within the recommended range as they varied between 6.6 and 7.7. Compliance with the standard was also observed for saturation with oxygen (64.5–98.3%). Conductivity of water (40.3–77.2 mS/m) is directly related to the concentration of salts dissolved in water. The level of this parameter was lower than in Sources 1 and 2, so were also the values of oxidisability COD_{Mn}, which ranged from 0.16 to 0.8 mg/L. These values indicated very low level of chemically oxidisable pollutants, and therefore low possibility of development of disinfection BPs at chlorination.

When disinfecting water with active chlorine, the level of chemical oxygen demand (COD) or oxidisability is very important. COD is a measure of the capacity of **water** to consume oxygen during the **decomposition** of organic **matter** and the oxidation of inorganic chemicals, such as ammonia and nitrite. Thus, it indicates potential risk of development of BPs, such as THMs and haloacetic acid, which are linked to increased risk of cancer [26, 27]. When assessing the vulnerability of groundwater, there is an assumption that the water closer to the soil surface is of greater risk of contamination by pollutants, including N compounds. The proportion of N forms in groundwater is also affected by the depth [57].

Nitrites and ammonium ions were not detected in Source 3 and nitrates ranged between 25 and 32 mg/L and only at one sampling exceeded the limit by 8 mg/L. Chloride levels persisted well below the limit of 250 mg/L (6.8–22.3 mg/L). The sum of calcium and magnesium in water from Source 3 ranged between 2.0 and 2.4 mmol/L, which was in the recommended range.

3.3. EEM fluorescence spectra of water from Sources 1 to 3

Contamination of treated drinking water may occur while passing through the distribution system consumers. Elevated levels of dissolved organic matter (DOM) by the consumer compared to the water leaving the treatment plant indicates potential contamination that can be measured sensitively, inexpensively, and potentially online via fluorescence and absorbance spectroscopy. However, we lack the knowledge how much natural variation can be expected in a stable distribution system [58].

DOM plays an essential role in biogeochemical cycles and in transport of organic matter throughout the hydrological continuum. Fox et al. [59] used excitation-emission matrix (EEM) fluorescence spectroscopy to characterise microbially derived organic matter from common environmental microorganisms (*E. coli, Bacillus subtilis,* and *P. aeruginosa*). Their study showed that bacterial organisms can produce fluorescent organic matter (FOM) in situ and, furthermore, that the production of FOM differs at a bacterial species level. Fluorescence spectroscopy is a reliable and highly sensitive optical technique that allows one to carry out rapid monitoring of DOM in both natural and engineered systems. Fluorescence excitation emission matrices (EEMs) provide plenty of information about DOM [60].

EEM indicates the presence of pollutants by means of fluorescence characteristics, namely position of fluorophore in EEM, or excitation and emission maximum. Recent studies showed that different ways of disinfection of water affect its fluorescence properties due to development of various disinfection BPs [61]. The basis for correct evaluation of EEM of respective samples is the determination of a standard that can be used for comparison of quality at the absence of previous chemical analysis. Sample of drinking water taken from public drinking water supply (**Figure 1**) was used as a graphic standard in our study.

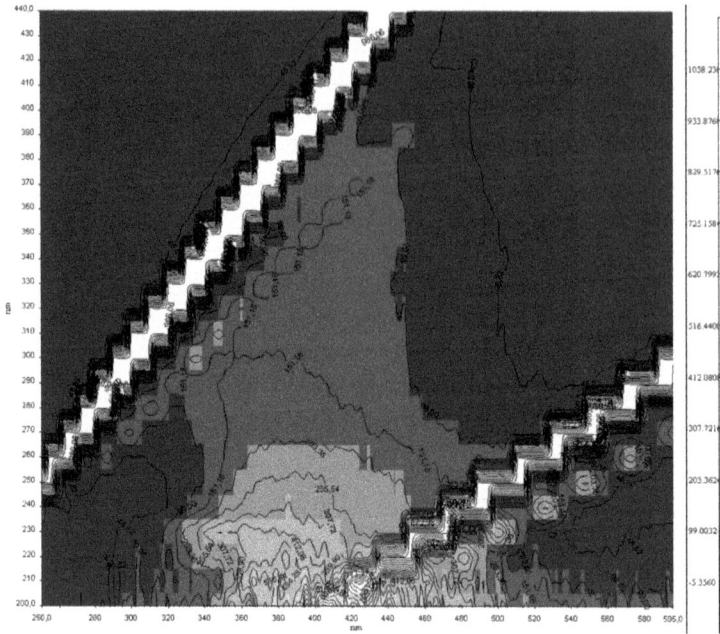

Figure 1. EEM of potable water sample from public water main.

4. Conclusion

Physico-chemical, microbiological examination, and EEM fluorescence spectroscopy used to investigate water from three monitored sources showed that the Source 3 provided water of better quality than Sources 1 and 2 (**Figures 2–4**). The results obtained did not indicate pollution of water with animal or human wastes. Some discrepancies between results of EEM spectroscopy and other analyses could be explained by limited number of EEM examinations and inability to identify the sources of NOM detected by this method.

Our results also suggested that weather (precipitations) was most likely the reason why quality of water was adversely affected at some samplings. The presence of total coliform bacteria indicated potential risk to animals consuming this water. However, according to some sources, total coliform testing can detect bacteria that have no connection with faecal contamination. Also, results of physico-chemical examination did not indicate faecal pollution. This is a complex issue requiring additional more detailed investigations.

The dose of chloramine-T determined by experimental chlorination and used for disinfection of investigated sources appeared effective only for Source 3, while they have to be doubled for Sources 1 and 2, and even these increased doses were much lower than the dose recommended by the manufacturer of this preparation. This is important from the point of view of decreasing production of potential BPs of water disinfection with active chlorine preparation. It may be more appropriate to adjust the intervals between individual treatments (disinfection) to weather conditions (heavy rain) instead of significantly increasing the active chlorine doses.

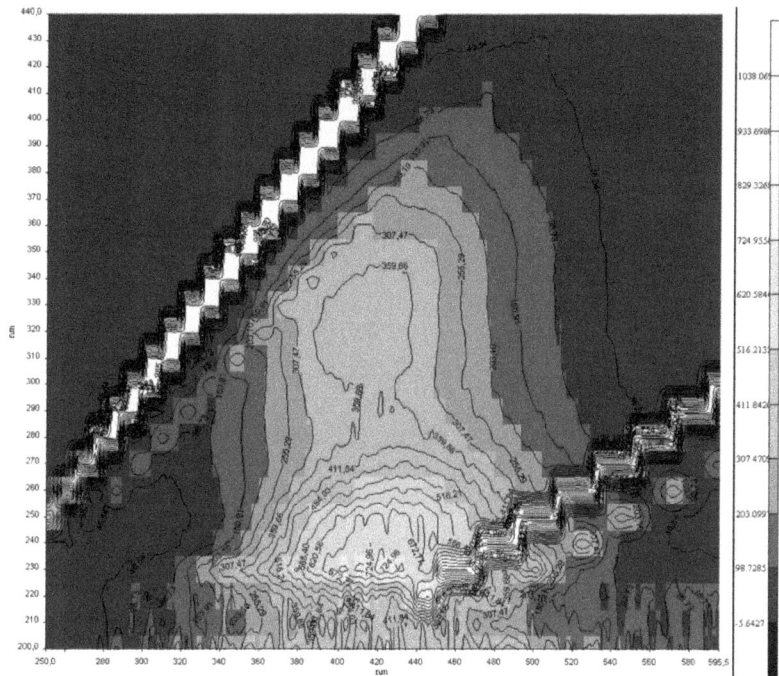

Figure 2. EEM of water sample of Source 1.

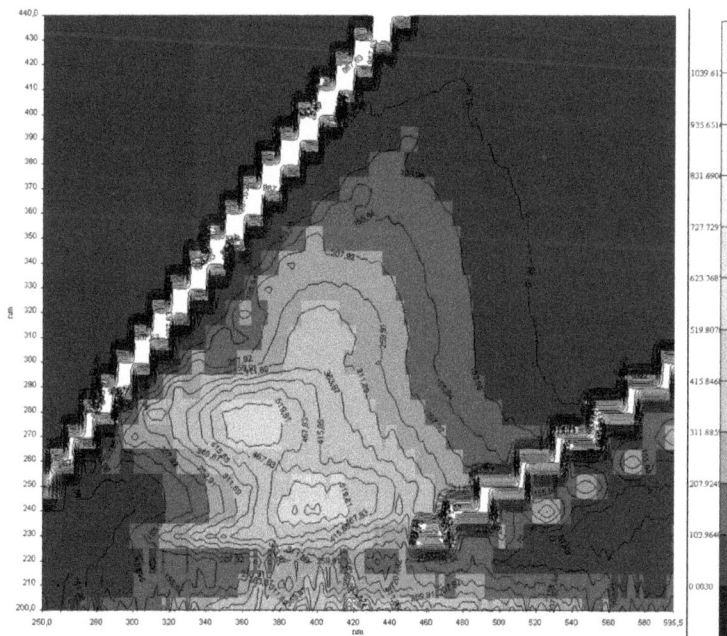

Figure 3. EEM of water sample of Source 2.

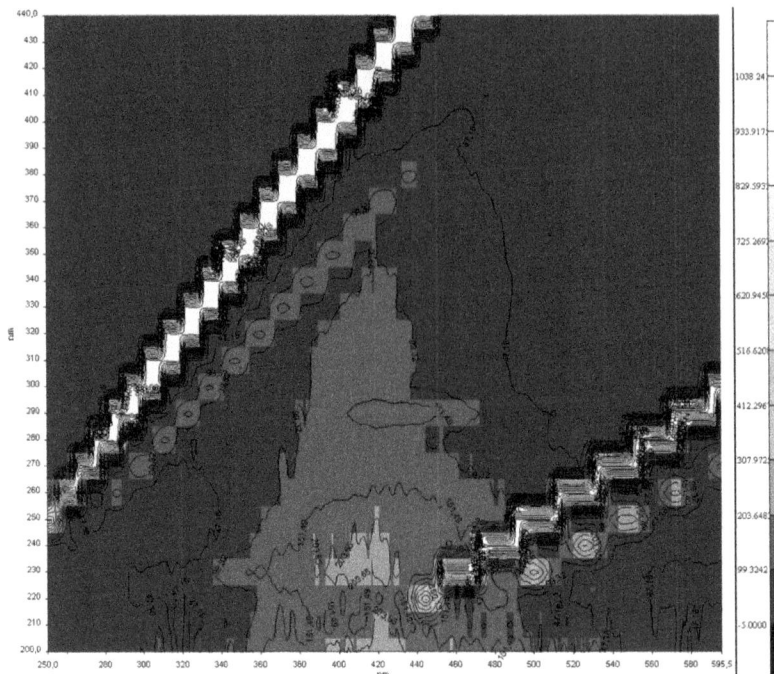

Figure 4. EEM of water sample of Source 3.

Acknowledgements

The study was supported by the project VEGA 2/0125/17 and Slovak Ministry of Culture and Education Grant Agency No. 003UVLF-4/2016.

Author details

Tatiana Hrušková[1]*, Naďa Sasáková[2], Gabriela Gregová[2], Ingrid Papajová[3] and Zuzana Bujdošová[1]

*Address all correspondence to: tatiana.hruskova@uvlf.sk

1 Department of Chemistry, Biochemistry and Biophysics, Institute of Medical Chemistry, University of Veterinary Medicine and Pharmacy in Košice, Košice, Slovak Republic

2 Department of Environment, Veterinary Legislation and Economy, University of Veterinary Medicine and Pharmacy in Košice, Košice, Slovak Republic

3 Parasitological Institute of the Slovak Academy of Sciences, Košice, Slovak Republic

References

[1] WHO. Guidelines for Drinking-water Quality: Incorporating 1st and 2nd Addenda. Recommendations. 3rd ed. Geneva: World Health Organization; 2008. p. 1

[2] Regulation of the government of the SR No. 368/2007 Coll. on protection of farm animals, part 162, page 2670, [Internet]. 2007. Available from: http://www.svssr.sk/dokumenty/legislativa/nv_368_2007.pdf [Accessed: Dec 10-2017]

[3] Act No. 322/2003 Coll. on protection of farm animals, specifying that all sources of water used for watering of animals must comply with the requirements on water intended for human consumption, part 146, page 2604, [Internet]. 2003. Available from: http://www.svssr.sk/dokumenty/legislativa/nv_322_2003.pdf [Accessed: Dec 12-2017]

[4] Slovak Republic Government Order Act No. 496/2010 Coll. defining requirements for water intended for human consumption and quality control of water intended for human consumption, part 188, page 4207, [Internet]. 2010. Available from: http://www.ecoli.sk/files/documents/nv_496_2010.pdf [Accessed: Dec 10-2017]

[5] Fawell J, Nieuwenhuijsen JM. Contaminants in drinking water: Environmental pollution and health. British Medical Bulletin. 2003;**68**:199-208. DOI: 10.1093/bmb/ldg027

[6] Adams B, Foster SSD. Land-surface zoning for groundwater protection. Water and Environment Journal. 1992;**6**:312-319. DOI: 10.1111/j.1747-6593.1992.tb00755.x

[7] EPA. Water Treatment Manual: Disinfection, Environmental Protection Agency. Wexford, Ireland: Johnstown Castle Co; 2011. 187 p. ISBN: 978-184095-421-0

[8] Fridrich B, Krčmar D, Dalmacija B, Molnar J, Pešić V, Kragulj M, Varga N. Impact of wastewater from pig farm lagoons on the quality of local groundwater. Agricultural Water and Management. 2014;**135**:40-53. DOI: 10.1016/j.agwat.2013.12.014

[9] Sasakova N, Veselitz-Lakticova K, Hromada R, Chvojka D, Kosco J, Ondrasovic M. Contamination of individual sources of drinking water located in environmentally polluted central Spis region (Slovakia). Journal of Microbiology, Biotechnology and Food Sciences. 2013;**3**(3):262-265

[10] Directive 2010/75/EU of the European Parliament and of the Council on industrial emissions (integrated pollution prevention and control), Official Journal of the European Union, L 334/17, [Internet]. 2010. Available from: https://eur-lex.europa.eu/legal-content/EN/TXT/?uri=celex%3A32010L0075 [Accessed: Dec 10-2017]

[11] WHO: Guidelines for Drinking-water Quality. Health Criteria and Other Supporting Information. 2nd ed. Geneva: World Health Organization; 1996. p. 2

[12] WHO: Hardness in Drinking-water. Background Document for Preparation of WHO Guidelines for Drinking-water Quality. Geneva: World Health Organization (WHO/HSE/WSH/10.01/10/Rev/1). 2011. 19 p

[13] Leclerc H, Mossel DAA, Edberg SC, Struijk CB. Advances in the bacteriology of the coli-form group: Their suitability as markers of microbial water safety. Annual Review of Microbiology. 2001;**55**:201-234. DOI: 10.1146/annurev.micro.55.1.201

[14] Cabral JPS. Water microbiology. Bacterial pathogens and water. International Journal of Environmental Research and Public Health. 2010;**7**:3657-3703. DOI: 10.3390/ijerph7103657

[15] Pitter P. Hydrochemie (in Czech). 4th ed. Prague: VŠCHT; 2009. 568 p. (Edited book)

[16] Block SS, editor. Disinfection, Sterilization and Preservation. 5th ed. Philadelphia: Lippincott Williams & Wilkins; 2001. 1485 p. ISBN: 0-683-30740-1

[17] Macler AB, Pontius WF. Groundwater disinfection: Chlorine's role in public health. Journal American Water Works Association. 1997;**4**

[18] Sasakova N, Vargova M, Gregova G. Protection of the Environment and Public Health. 1st ed. Košice: UVLF; 2014. 217 p. ISBN: 978-80-8077-435-6

[19] Kijovska L. The effects of disinfectants on microorganisms. In: Kijovska L, editors. Ecotoxi-cology in Slovak Water Management (in Slovak). 1st ed. Bratislava: STU; 2013. pp. 234-236

[20] Gunten U. Ozonation of drinking water: Part II. Disinfection and by-product forma-tion in presence of bromide, iodide or chlorine. Water Research. 2003;**37**:1469-1487. DOI: 10.1016/S0043-1354(02)00458-X

[21] Sorlini S, Gialdini F, Biasibetti M, Collivignarelli C. Influence of drinking water treat-ments on chlorine dioxide consumption and chlorite/chlorate formation. Water Research. 2014;**54**:44-52. DOI: 10.1016/j.watres.2014.01.038

[22] Schmidt LJ, Gaikowski MP, Gingerich WH, Stehly GR, Larson WJ, Dawson VK, Schreier TM. Environmental Assessment of the Effects of Chloramine-T Use in and Discharge by Freshwater Aquaculture. Submitted to U.S. Food and Drug Administration Center for Veterinary Medicine Director, Division of Therapeutic Drugs for Food Animals Office of New Animal Drug Evaluation, Maryland. April 2007. 136 p

[23] Gottardi W. Aqueous chloramine T solutions as disinfectants: chemical composition, reactivity and toxicity (Article in German). Archiv der Pharmazie (Weinheim). 1992;**325**: 377-384

[24] Cipriano RC, Ford LA, Starliper CE, Teska JD, Nelson JT, Jensen BN. Control of external *Aeromonas salmonicida*: Topical disinfection of Salmonids with Chloramine-T. Journal of Aquatic Animal Health. 1996;**8**:52-57. DOI: 10.1577/1548-8667(1996)008<0052:COEAST>2.3.CO;2

[25] Bessems E. Bactericidal Effect of Halamid® According to the CEN Test for Application in Food, Industrial, Domestic and Institutional Areas. Report submitted by the Department of Microbiology of AKZO Nobel Central Research, Duren. August 15, 1996; Duren. 5 p

[26] Chowdhury S. Exposure assessment for trihalomethanes in municipal drinking water and risk reduction strategy. Science of the Total Environment. 2013;**463/464**:922-930. DOI: 10.1016/j.scitotenv.2013.06.104

[27] Lyon AB, Cory MR, Weinberg SH. Changes in dissolved organic matter fluorescence and disinfection byproduct formation from UV and subsequent chlorination/chloramination. Journal of Hazardous Materials. 2013;**264**:411-419. DOI: 10.11949/j.issn.0438-1157.20141708

[28] Zhao YA, Anichina JA, Lu XA, Bull RJ, Krasner SC, Hrudey ES, Li X. Occurrence and formation of chloro- and bromobenzoquinones during drinking water disinfection. Water Research. 2012;**46**:4351-4360. DOI: 10.1016/j.watres.2012.05.032

[29] Horakova M, Lischke P, Grünwald A. Water Analytics. 1st ed. Prague: VŠCHT; 2003. 335 p. (in Czech)

[30] Jirotkova D, Soch M, Kernerova V, Palka V, Eidelpesova L. Use of electrolyzed water in animal production. Journal of Microbiology, Biotechnology and Food Sciences. 2012;**2**: 447-483

[31] Hussain SN, de las Heras N, Ashgar HM, Brown NW, Roberts EP. Disinfection of water by adsorption combined with electrochemical treatment. Water Research. 2014;**54**:170-178. DOI: 10.1016/j.watres.2014.01.043

[32] Li M, Qiang Z, Bolton J, Li W, Chen P. UV disinfection of secondary water supply: Online monitoring with micro-fluorescent silica detectors. Chemical Engineering Journal. 2014;**255**:165-170. DOI: 10.1016/j.cej.2014.06.025

[33] Sila ON, Kotut K, Okemo P. Techniques for potable water treatment using appropriate low cost natural materials in the tropics. Journal of Microbiology, Biotechnology and Food Sciences. 2013;**2**(5):2294-2300

[34] Liu W, Zhang Z, Yang X, Xu Y, Liang Y. Effects of UV irradiation and UV/chlorine co-exposure on natural organic matter in water. Science of the Total Environment. 2012;**414**:576-584. DOI: 10.1016/j.scitotenv.2011.11.031

[35] Raudales R, Parke J, Guy LCh, Fisher RP. Control of waterborne microbes in irrigation: A review. Agricultural Water Management. 2014;**143**:9-28. DOI: 10.1016/j.agwat.2014.06.007

[36] Hruskova T, Sasakova N, Bujdosova Z, Kvokacka V, Gregova G, Verebova V, Valko-Rokytovska M, Takac L. Disinfection of potable water sources on animal farms and their microbiological safety. Veterinarni Medicina. 2016;**61**:73-186. DOI: 10.17221/8818-VETMED

[37] Michalus M, Bratska Z. Medical-sanitary requirements for drinking water in light of current legislation in the Slovak Republic (in Slovak). Groundwater. 2000;**6**(2):59-66. ISSN: 1335-1052

[38] Ashbolt JN. Microbial contamination of drinking water and disease outcomes in developing regions. Toxicology. 2004;**198**:229-238. DOI: 10.1016/j.tox.2004.01.030

[39] Varchola V, Kijovský P, Kijovský F. Agrofarma Kijovsky – The largest producer of Fleckvieh bulls for natural mating in Slovakia. Fleckviehworld. 2013/2014:35-37

[40] STN EN ISO 9308-1. Water quality. Enumeration of Escherichia coli and coliform bacteria. Part 1: Membrane filtration method for waters with low bacterial background flora,

[Internet]. 2015. Available from: https://www.sutn.sk/eshop/public/standard_detail. aspx?id=121405 [Accessed:J Dec 10-2017]

[41] STN EN ISO 7899-2. Water quality. Detection and enumeration of intestinal entero-cocci. Part 2: Membrane filtration method (ISO 7899-2:2000) [Internet]. 2000. Available from: https://www.sutn.sk/eshop/public/standard_detail.aspx?id=91499 [Accessed: Dec 10-2017]

[42] EC Regulations. European Communities (Drinking Water) Regulations, Statutory Instruments No. 106 of 2007. [Internet]. 2007. Available from: https://www.fsai.ie/upload-edFiles/Legislation/Food_Legisation_Links/Water/S.I_No_06_of_2007.pdf   [Accessed: Dec 10-2017]

[43] Bochemie. Production for Schulke [Internet]. 2015. Available from: https://www.boche-mie.cz/en/cleaning-and-disinfecting-agents/about-private-labels#kategorie [Accessed: Dec 10, 2017]

[44] STN ISO 9297. Water quality. Determination of chloride. Silver nitrate titration with chromate indicator (Mohr's method) [Internet]. 2000. Available from: https://www.sutn. sk/eshop/public/standard_detail.aspx?id=79117 [Accessed: Dec 12-2017]

[45] STN EN ISO 7393-3. Water quality. Determination of free chlorine and total chlorine. Part 3: Iodometric titration method for the determination of total chlorine [Internet]. 2001. Available from: https://www.sutn.sk/eshop/public/standard_detail.aspx?id=79116 [Accessed: Dec 10-2017]

[46] STN EN ISO 5814. Water quality. Determination of dissolved oxygen. Electrochemical probe method [Internet]. 2013. Available from: https://www.sutn.sk/eshop/public/stan-dard_detail.aspx?id=117106 [Accessed: Dec 12-2017]

[47] STN EN ISO 8467. Water quality. Determination of permanganate index [Internet]. 2000. Available from: https://www.sutn.sk/eshop/public/standard_detail.aspx?id=79124 [Accessed: Dec 10-2017]

[48] Dubayova K, Ticha M, Kusnir J, Luckova I, Rigdova K, Gondova T. The fluorescence contour map as "identity card" of spring waters (in Slovak). Book of Abstracts of the Conference The Use of Chemical Methods in Protecting and Promoting Public Health; September 9-10, 2008; LF UPJŠ Košice. 2008. p.13

[49] Ojo IO, Otieno OAF, Ochieng MG. Groundwater: Characteristics, qualities, pollu-tions and treatments: An overview. International Journal of Water Resources and Environmental Engineering. 2012;4:162-170. DOI: 10.5897/IJWREE12.038

[50] Badawy MI, Gad-Allah TA, Ali EMM, Yoon Y. Minimization of the formation of disinfec-tion by-products. Chemosphere. 2012;89:235-240. DOI: 10.1016/j.chemosphere. 2012.04.025

[51] Bonton A, Rouleau A, Bouchard C, Rodriguez JM. Assessment of groundwater qual-ity and its variations in the capture zone of a pumping well in an agricultural area. Agricultural Water Management. 2010;97:824-834. DOI: 10.1016/j.agwat.2010.01.009

[52] Cho CJ, Cho BH, Kim JS. Heavy contamination of a subsurface aquifer and a stream by livestock wastewater in a stock farming area, Wonju, Korea. Environmental Pollution. 1999;**109**:137-146. DOI: 10.1016/S0269-7491(99)00230-4

[53] Environmental Health Fact Sheet (EHFS). Chemical aspects. chap. 8 Available from: http://search.who.int/search?q=chlorination+with+HOCl+-+pH&ie=utf8&site=who&client=_en_r&proxystylesheet=_en_r&output=xml_no_dtd&oe=utf8&getfields=doctype [Accessed: Dec 10-2017]

[54] Bartel-Hunt S, Snow DD, Damon-Powell T, Miesbach D. Occurrence of steroid hormones and antibiotics in shallow groundwater impacted by livestock waste control facilities. Journal of Contaminant Hydrology. 2011;**123**:94-103. DOI: 10.1016/j.jconhyd.2010.12.010

[55] Kroupova H, Machova J, Svobodova Z. Nitrite influence on fish: A review. Veterinární Medicína. 2005;**50**:461-471

[56] Krapac IG, Dey WS, Roy WR, Smyth CA, Storment E, Sargent SL, Steele JD. Impacts of swine manure pits on groundwater quality. Environmental Pollution. 2002;**120**:475-492. DOI: 10.1016/S0269-7491(02)00115-X

[57] Morari F, Lugato E, Polese R, Berti A, Giardini L. Nitrate concentrations in groundwater under contrasting agricultural management practices in the low plains of Italy. Agriculture, Ecosystems and Environment. 2012;**147**:17-56. DOI: 10.1016/j.agee.2011.03.001

[58] Heibati M, Stedmon CA, Stenroth K, Rauch S, Toljander J, Säve-Söderbergh M, Murphy KR. Assessment of drinking water quality at the tap using fluorescence spectroscopy. Water Research. 2017;**125**:1-10. DOI: 10.1016/j.watres.2017.08.020

[59] Fox BG, Thorn RMS, Anesio AM, Reynolds DM. The *in situ* bacterial production of fluorescent organic matter; an investigation at a species level. Water Research. 2017;**125**:350-359. DOI: 10.1016/j.watres.2017.08.040

[60] Yang L, Hur J, Zhuang W. Occurrence and behaviors of fluorescence EEM-PARAFAC components in drinking water and wastewater treatment systems and their applications: A review. Environmental Science and Pollution Research. 2015;**22**:6500-6510. DOI: 10.1007/s11356-015-4214-3

[61] Markechova D, Tomkova M, Sadecka J. Fluorescence excitation – Emission matrix spectroscopy and parallel factor analysis in drinking water treatment: A review. Polish Journal of Environmental Studies. 2013;**22**:1289-1295

Viral Disinfection

Chapter 3

Carrier and Liquid Heat Inactivation of Poliovirus and Adenovirus

S. Steve Zhou, Cameron Wilde, Zheng Chen,
Tanya Kapes, Jennifer Purgill, Raymond Nims and
Donna Suchmann

Additional information is available at the end of the chapter

http://dx.doi.org/10.5772/intechopen.76340

Abstract

Viral inactivation is typically studied using virus suspended in liquid (liquid inactivation) or virus deposited on surfaces (carrier inactivation). Carrier inactivation more closely mimics disinfection of virus contaminating a surface, while liquid inactivation mimics virus inactivation in process solutions. The prevailing opinion has been that viruses are more susceptible to heat inactivation when suspended in liquid than when deposited on surfaces. In part, this reflects a paucity of comparative studies performed in a side-by-side manner. In the present study, we investigated the relative susceptibilities of the enteroviruses poliovirus-1 and adenovirus type 5 to heat inactivation in liquid versus carrier studies. The results of our side-by-side studies suggest that these two viruses are more readily inactivated when heat is applied to virus deposited on carriers. Decimal reduction values (i.e., the amount of time required to reduce the virus titer by one $\log_{10}$) measured at 46°C displayed the greatest difference between carrier and liquid inactivation approaches, with values ranging from 14.0 to 15.2 min (carrier) and from 47.4 to 64.1 min (liquid) for poliovirus. The corresponding values for adenovirus 5 were 18.2–29.2 min (carrier) and 20.8–38.3 min (liquid). At 65°C, the decimal reduction values were more similar (from 4 to 6 min) for the various inactivation approaches.

Keywords: adenovirus, carrier inactivation, enterovirus, liquid inactivation, poliovirus, thermal inactivation

1. Introduction

Heat (thermal) inactivation is one of several physical approaches that may be employed to inactivate viruses suspended in solutions or deposited on surfaces. Unlike chemical inactivation approaches that often display greater efficacy for lipid-enveloped viruses than for nonenveloped viruses, heat inactivation has been found to display effectiveness for both enveloped and nonenveloped viruses [1]. Heating appears to open the viral capsid, exposing the genomic material to nucleases present in the immediate environment [2, 3]. Therefore, the capsid conformation appears to be the main determinant of heat inactivation susceptibility [3, 4], not the envelope status.

In the past, heat inactivation has more typically been evaluated in liquid inactivation studies. In these studies, a solution of known virus titer is heated at a given temperature for a given amount of time and the final titer is measured (**Scheme 1**). A decimal reduction value (D) in units of time required for one $\log_{10}$ decrease in titer is then calculated. Such studies are appropriate when evaluating the effectiveness of inactivation processes aimed at virus infectivity reduction in solutions (e.g., pasteurization). When the susceptibility of viruses deposited on a surface to heating is to be evaluated, such studies are most appropriately performed using carriers (**Scheme 1**) [5, 6]. A known amount of virus is applied to the carriers (small representative pieces of a given material type) and allowed to dry in the absence or presence of a matrix (such as blood, saline, or culture medium). After a given drying time, the carriers and virus deposited thereon are subjected to a given duration of heating at a given temperature. The remaining infectious virus is recovered from the carriers and is measured and, again, a $\log_{10}$ reduction value and corresponding D value may be determined.

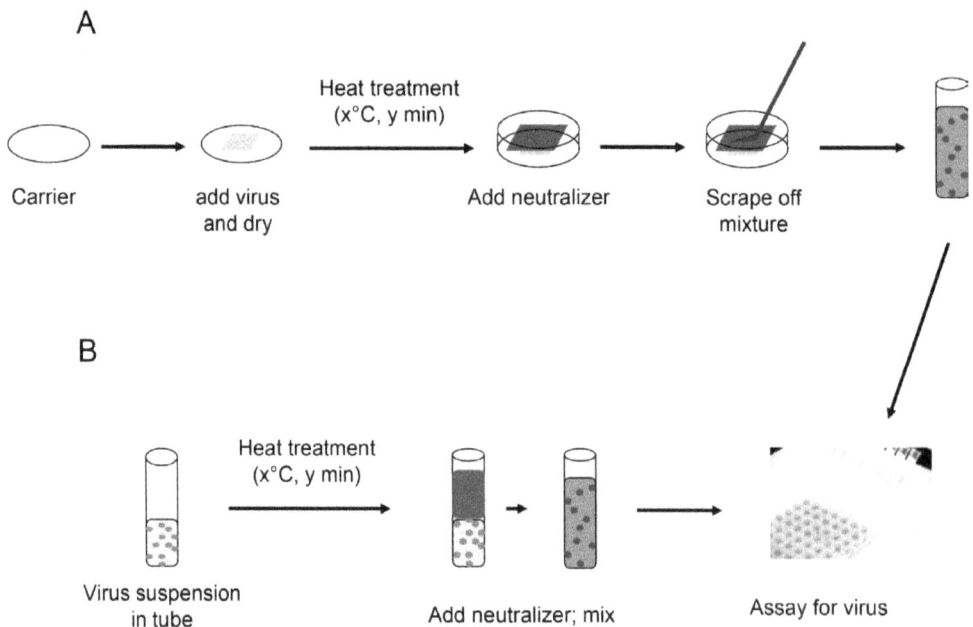

Scheme 1. High-level flow diagrams for carrier (A) and liquid (B) inactivation study design.

There have been relatively few studies that have evaluated heat inactivation of viruses on carriers [5–11], and we are aware of only a single study directly comparing liquid and carrier heat inactivation in a side-by-side format [11]. The prevailing opinion has been that viruses are more susceptible to heating in liquid than when deposited on surfaces and that dry heat efficacy is related to residual moisture or relative humidity [7, 9–12]. In order to clarify the relative susceptibilities of model enteroviruses to liquid and carrier inactivation, we have evaluated poliovirus-1 (PV-1; family Picornaviridae) and adenovirus type 5 (Ad5; family Adenoviridae) inactivation in two liquid matrices (medium containing 5% serum [medium] or undiluted fetal bovine serum [serum]) or when deposited on two carrier materials (stainless steel [Steel] or glass). The two enteroviruses may be transmitted by the fecal-oral route and therefore ability to inactivate viruses dried onto surfaces following deposition from contaminated water is of public health interest. See **Box 1** for information about poliovirus, adenovirus and associated disease.

Box 1. Poliovirus, adenovirus, and associated disease. The majority of PV-1 infections result in an abortive flu-like prodrome or are asymptomatic. In ~5% of infections, a meningitic phase follows the prodrome as the virus displays a predilection for the nervous system [13]. Spinal poliomyelitis with varying degrees of flaccid weakness follows shortly in some cases, while a bulbar form with minimal limb involvement but higher mortality can also occur. Interestingly, the "summer plague" of poliomyelitis that was experienced between 1916 and the advent of vaccination in the mid-1950s has been attributed in part to improvements in community sanitation [13] occurring around the turn of the century. The herd immunity that previously existed due to early infection coinciding with presence of maternal antibodies was lost when sanitation improved. Acquisition of the infection later in childhood was associated with a greater chance for poliomyelitis. Poliomyelitis still occurs in certain underdeveloped regions of the world, despite efforts at global eradication.

Adenoviruses can cause respiratory and gastrointestinal infections. Adenovirus types 40 and 41 represent common cases of infantile gastroenteritis, although most of the 41 types of adenovirus may be recovered from the feces of patients. These enteroviruses may be spread by the fecal-oral route. Contamination of water supplies and fomites (environmental surfaces) can lead to transmission of the enteritis from infected to noninfected individuals [14].

---

2. Materials and methods

2.1. Viruses

Poliovirus type 1 (PV-1), strain Chat, was propagated in rhesus monkey kidney LLC-MK2 derivative cells (American Type Culture Collection CCL-7.1). The virus was diluted in Roswell Park Memorial Institute (RPMI) medium supplemented with 5% newborn calf serum (NCS, source: ThermoFisher Scientific, Waltham, MA) and added to T-75 flasks of the LLC-MK2 cells. The flasks were incubated at $36 \pm 2°C$ with $5 \pm 1\%$ CO_2 for 90 min to allow for viral adsorption, after which they were refed with growth medium. Incubation was continued at $36 \pm 2°C$ with $5 \pm 1\%$ CO_2 until 90% of the cells exhibited viral cytopathic effect (CPE). The flasks were frozen at −80°C and then thawed at room temperature. The medium from the flasks was collected and clarified by centrifugation at 2000 rpm for 15 min and the resulting supernatant was aliquoted and stored at −80°C until use. The certified titer of the stock PV-1 was determined to be 6.79 $\log_{10}$ tissue culture infective dose$_{50}$ per mL (TCID$_{50}$/mL) in MA-104 cells (Charles River Laboratories, Germantown, MD).

Adenovirus type 5 (Ad5), strain Adenoid 75, was propagated in human lung epithelial A549 cells (American Type Culture Collection CCL-185). The virus was diluted in Dulbecco's Modified Eagle Medium (DMEM) supplemented with 5% fetal bovine serum (FBS, source: ThermoFisher Scientific, Waltham, MA) and added to T-75 flasks of the A549 cells. The flasks were incubated at 36 ± 2°C with 5 ± 1% CO_2 for 90 min to allow for viral adsorption, after which they were refed with the growth medium. Incubation was continued at 36 ± 2°C with 5 ± 1% CO_2 until 100% of the cells exhibited viral CPE. The flasks were frozen at −80°C and then thawed at room temperature. The medium from the flasks was collected and clarified by centrifugation at 2000 rpm for 15 min and the resulting supernatant was aliquoted and stored at −80°C until use. The certified titer of the stock Ad5 virus stock was determined to be 7.01 $\log_{10}$ TCID$_{50}$/mL in A549 cells.

2.2. Carriers and liquid matrices

Glass carriers consisted of 4-in^2 area of a sterile glass Petri dish. Steel carriers consisted of brushed stainless steel discs of 1 cm in diameter. The serum matrix consisted of undiluted FBS, while the medium matrix consisted of RPMI medium containing 5% NCS for PV-1 and DMEM medium containing 5% FBS for Ad5.

2.3. Evaluation of heat inactivation (duplicate replicates)

Virus was spread onto the glass carriers (0.4 mL virus suspension) or steel carriers (0.05 mL virus suspension) and allowed to dry at room temperature (20–21°C) per ASTM International (ASTM) standard E1053 [15]. For liquid inactivation, 0.2 mL of virus suspension was added to 1.8 mL of serum or medium in glass tubes per ASTM standard E1052 [16].

Carriers containing virus were placed into a hot-air oven (Isotemp™ General Purpose, Fisher Scientific Catalog No. 151030509) set at one of three test temperatures (46, 56 and 65°C) for 5, 20, or 60 min. The relative humidity of the oven was not measured.

Glass tubes containing virus/medium or virus/serum solutions prepared as described earlier were placed into a hot air oven set at one of three test temperatures (46, 56 and 65°C) for 5, 20, or 60 min. The relative humidity of the oven was not measured.

Following the heating times, 4 mL of neutralizer (FBS) was added to the virus film on the glass or steel carriers and used to remove the film from the surface with cell scrapers. The liquid heat inactivation conditions were neutralized following heating by addition of 2 mL of cold neutralizer.

Post-neutralization samples were serially diluted and selected dilutions were inoculated onto the proper host cells for each virus (8-wells per dilution in 96-well plates). A virus recovery control (VRC) was included to determine the relative loss in virus infectivity as a result of drying and neutralization. Virus was applied to the carriers (glass or steel) or added to liquids (serum or medium) and held at room temperature ($20 \pm 1°C$) for the longest contact time evaluated (60 min). The resulting $TCID_{50}$/mL titer results for the VRC were then compared to heat-treated titers for the corresponding carrier/matrix type to calculate the reduction in infectivity caused by heat treatment. The various 96-well plates were incubated at $36 \pm 2°C$ with $5 \pm 1\%$ CO_2 for 6–9 days (PV-1) or 11–14 days (Ad5). Following incubation, the plates were scored for CPE. The 50% tissue culture infective dose per mL ($TCID_{50}$/mL) was calculated using the Spearman-Kärber formula [17].

2.4. Calculation of D and z values and power function analysis

Decimal reduction (D) values were estimated from the most linear portions of the inactivation versus time curves for the various set temperatures (not shown). The plots included both replicate values for any given temperature and time point, therefore represent an analysis of the pooled replicate data, with a single D value being generated. Rapid deviation from linearity in these plots was noted as complete inactivation of virus occurred rapidly at the higher temperatures. We acknowledge that a certain degree of error is associated with the D value estimation process. Such errors do not detract from the validity of the comparisons to be made between carrier and liquid inactivation results, since comparison of the raw inactivation versus time results obtained leads to similar conclusions.

The z value (°C per $\log_{10}$ change in D) for a given data set was obtained from plots of $\log_{10}D$ versus temperature (not shown), evaluated using the linear regression function of Excel. The z value is obtained as 1/slope (m) from the linear fit equation (Eq. (1)):

$$y = mx + b \tag{1}$$

where y = $\log_{10}D$, x = temperature, m = slope and b = y-axis intercept.

Plots of D versus temperature were evaluated using the power function of Excel to obtain the line fit equation (Eq. (2)):

$$y = ax^{-b} \tag{2}$$

where y = D, x = temperature and a and b are constants unique to each line fit equation. This equation allows one to extrapolate the D value at any given inactivation temperature and can also be rearranged to solve for temperature, as shown in (Eq. (3)).

$$temperature \ (°C) = \left(\frac{D}{a}\right)^{-\frac{1}{b}} \tag{3}$$

allowing one to estimate the inactivation temperature required to achieve a desired D value [18] (see also discussion later).

3. Results

3.1. Carrier and liquid heat inactivation results for PV-1

Replicate results for heat inactivation of PV-1 on carriers or in solutions are displayed in **Table 1**. Three exposure times (5, 20 and 60 min) and three temperatures (46, 56 and 65°C) were evaluated.

Mode	Inactivation matrix	Inactivation time (min)	Log_{10} reduction at inactivation temperature		
			46°C	56°C	65°C
Carrier inactivation					
	Glass	5	−0.25[a]	0.00	0.25
		5	−0.50	1.50	0.50
		20	−0.25	≥ 4.86	5.21
		20	0.00	≥ 5.72	≥ 5.10
		60	4.26	≥ 4.85	≥ 4.97
		60	4.71	≥ 5.72	≥ 5.10
	Steel	5	−0.25	0.25	0.25
		5	0.37	0.87	0.50
		20	1.63	≥ 4.97	≥ 4.72
		20	1.37	≥ 5.22	≥ 4.85
		60	≥ 4.35	≥ 4.97	≥ 4.72
		60	≥ 4.22	≥ 5.22	≥ 4.85
Liquid inactivation					
	Medium	5	0.00	0.00	0.12
		5	0.00	−0.13	0.75
		20	0.13	2.25	≥ 5.22
		20	0.13	2.12	≥ 5.60
		60	1.13	≥ 5.10	≥ 5.22
		60	0.88	≥ 4.22	≥ 5.60
	Serum	5	−0.25	0.37	0.00
		5	0.13	0.00	0.50
		20	0.00	2.12	≥ 5.22
		20	−0.12	2.00	5.38
		60	1.38	≥ 4.97	≥ 5.22
		60	1.50	≥ 4.35	≥ 5.47

[a]The values indicate the log_{10} reduction (log_{10} titer heated − log_{10} titer for VRC) for two replicates per time point. Values shown as "≥" indicate complete inactivation.

Table 1. Heat inactivation data for PV-1.

The results of a virus recovery control for the virus stock have been subtracted from the $\log_{10}$ reduction values displayed in this table. This corrects for any loss of infectivity associated with drying of the virus stock and recovery after a 1-h hold at room temperature. A striking difference in carrier versus liquid inactivation was noted for the 46°C study. The PV-1 heated on steel carriers was completely inactivated ($\geq$4.2 $\log_{10}$) in 60 min.

On glass carriers, 4.3–4.7 $\log_{10}$ PV-1 inactivation occurred in 60 min. During this time frame, less than 1.5 $\log_{10}$ inactivation of PV-1 occurred when liquid heating was compared. In the 56°C study, greater inactivation occurred on carriers by 20 min, compared to virus heated in solution. In the 65°C study, similar inactivation occurred for virus heated on carriers or in solution, regardless of the inactivation time.

In order to reduce the heat inactivation data for PV-1 to a form usable for comparisons between viruses and between matrices/carriers, D values (minutes required for 1 $\log_{10}$ titer reduction) were estimated from the most linear portions of the inactivation versus time curves for the various set temperatures. The D values, displayed in **Table 2**, were then used to generate $\log_{10}D$ versus temperature curves from which z values (°C per $\log_{10}$ change in D) were obtained. Plots of D versus temperature (**Figure 1**) depict a surface along which the D required for 1 $\log_{10}$ inactivation at any given heating temperature is displayed.

3.2. Carrier and liquid heat inactivation results for Ad5

Replicate results for heat inactivation of Ad5 on carriers and in solutions are shown in **Table 3**. These studies involved the same temperatures and exposure times used for the PV-1 studies described earlier. The $\log_{10}$ reduction values have again been corrected for the virus recovery control. In the case of Ad5, differences in susceptibility to heat inactivation on glass carriers, relative to steel carriers, were noted at each temperature, with greater inactivation at any

Temperature	D values (min)				
	Glass		Steel	Medium	Serum
46°C	15.2		14.0	64.1	47.4
56°C	3.9		4.1	12.5	10.1
65°C	4.0		4.4	3.9	9.3
	z values (°C per $\log_{10}$ change in D)				
	32		37	16	27
	Power function coefficients				
a	6 × 10⁷		8 × 10⁶	2 × 10¹⁵	5 × 10⁹
b	4.02		3.50	8.11	4.87

Table 2. Estimated D, z and power function values for PV-1.

exposure time being observed on steel carriers. In general, heat inactivation on carriers was found to be similar to that observed in solutions, with no clear differences noted between temperature dependence and time kinetics.

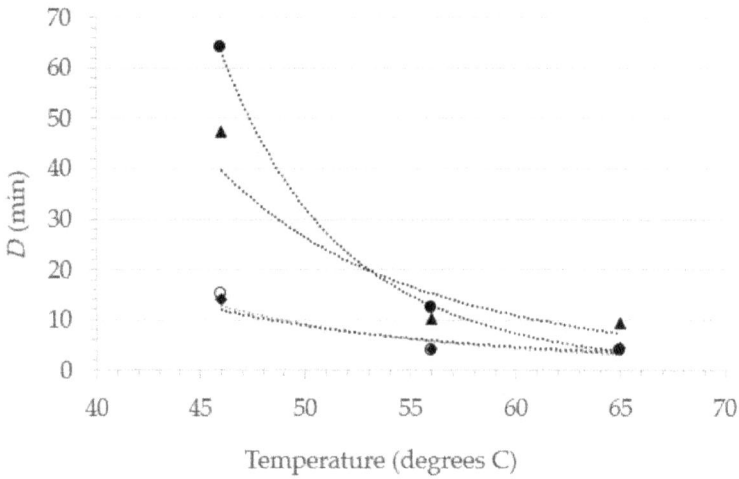

Figure 1. D vs. temperature relationships for heat inactivation of PV-1 on Steel (◆) or Glass (○) carriers and Medium (●) or Serum (▲) liquid matrices. All points along the fit lines represent 1 $\log_{10}$ inactivation of PV-1.

Mode	Inactivation matrix	Inactivation time (min)	Log_{10} reduction at inactivation temperature		
			46°C	56°C	65°C
Carrier inactivation					
	Glass	5	1.12[a]	1.25	1.63
		5	0.50	1.00	2.00
		20	2.00	1.63	2.88
		20	0.88	1.00	2.75
		60	2.37	4.85	≥4.10
		60	1.13	4.47	≥4.10
	Steel	5	0.62	−0.25	0.75
		5	0.88	−0.13	−0.37
		20	2.25	3.20	3.85
		20	1.63	3.12	3.10
		60	3.10	≥ 3.97	≥ 3.85
		60	2.86	≥ 4.22	≥ 3.10

Mode	Inactivation matrix	Inactivation time (min)	Log$_{10}$ reduction at inactivation temperature		
			46°C	56°C	65°C
Liquid inactivation					
	Medium	5	0.25	−0.12	0.63
		5	0.38	−0.25	−0.25
		20	0.37	1.13	4.10
		20	0.63	1.75	3.35
		60	1.37	4.10	≥ 4.10
		60	1.75	4.10	≥ 3.35
	Serum	5	0.50	−0.37	0.62
		5	0.63	0.25	0.25
		20	0.38	2.25	4.22
		20	1.00	1.25	3.85
		60	2.63	4.10	≥ 4.22
		60	3.25	4.35	≥ 4.85

[a]The values indicate the log$_{10}$ reduction (log$_{10}$ titer heated − log$_{10}$ titer for VRC) for two replicates per time point. Values shown as "≥" indicate complete inactivation.

Table 3. Heat inactivation data for Ad5.

Temperature	D values (min)				
	Glass		Steel	Medium	Serum
46°C	29.2		18.2	38.3	20.8
56°C	12.9		6.8	14.7	14.0
65°C	6.5		6.0	5.6	5.1
	z values (°C per log$_{10}$ change in D)				
	29		39	23	32
	Power function coefficients				
a	5 × 10^8		5 × 10^6	6 × 10^{10}	8 × 10^7
b	4.34		3.28	5.51	3.95

Table 4. Estimated D, z and power function values for Ad5.

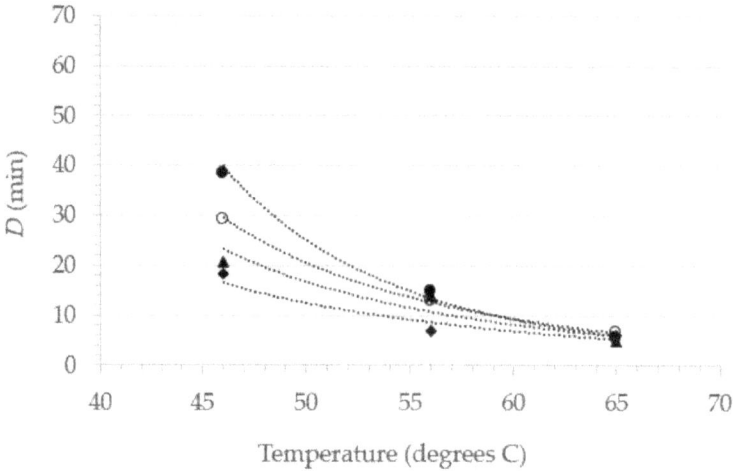

Figure 2. *D* vs. temperature relationships for heat inactivation of Ad5 on Steel (◆) or Glass (O) carriers and Medium (●) or Serum (▲) liquid matrices. All points along the fit lines represent 1 $\log_{10}$ inactivation of Ad5.

This conclusion may also be reached through examination of the calculated *D* and *z* values (**Table 4**) and the power function curves displaying the relationship between *D* and temperature (**Figure 2**). In no case was complete inactivation of the virus observed in exposure times under 60 min and with the exception of heating on steel carriers, complete inactivation was not observed at temperatures under 65°C.

4. Discussion of study results

A recent paradigm shift in virology has been the recognition of the important role of fomites (environmental porous and nonporous surfaces) in disseminating infectious virus (reviewed in [19, 20]). With this recognition has come a movement toward the conduct of carrier studies (in lieu of solution inactivation studies) to evaluate survival of viruses on typical fomite surfaces (glass, stainless steel, plastic, Formica, etc.) and to determine the efficacy of inactivation approaches for disinfection of contaminated fomites. This is not to say that carrier studies were not performed previously (e.g., [21]), but the literature for carrier inactivation of viruses was relatively sparse prior to the turn of the century. Arguments for and methodologies for conduct of carrier studies have become more common within the past two decades (e.g., [22, 23]) and a literature data base for viral inactivation on carriers is now accumulating. As mentioned within the introduction, however, side-by-side comparisons of inactivation efficacy in solutions versus on carriers are lacking. This is true in particular for thermal inactivation.

On the basis of the prevailing opinion [7, 9–12], our assumption going into these comparison studies was that we would confirm the expected increased resistance of viruses to dry heat inactivation as compared to heating in solutions. Although the humidity associated with carrier heating was not measured in our studies, this was expected to be low for a dry heat oven. This condition was predicted, on the basis of previous work [7, 11], to further reduce the effectiveness of the carrier heating approach, relative to liquid heating. Our side-by-side studies clearly did not confirm these expectations. For instance, PV-1 exhibited markedly reduced D values when subjected to dry heating at the relatively low temperature of 46°C, indicating increased susceptibility of this enterovirus, relative to liquid heating. This difference is not attributed to experimental artifact, since our liquid heating results compare reasonably well with previous results obtained for hepatitis A virus (another enterovirus from the Picornavirus family) inactivation in culture medium [24] and food homogenates [25, 26] (**Figure 3**; see also review by Bozkurt et al. [27]).

Our carrier results indicate a much greater sensitivity of PV-1 to dry heat than was determined by Sauerbrei and Wutzler [9]. These authors observed 4.3 $\log_{10}$ inactivation after 60 min at 75°C, providing an approximate D value of 13 min at this temperature. The differences may be due to methodology, as these authors also reported much different results for Ad5 relative to our results (see below). The impact of organic load on heat inactivation of PV-1 in our study was minimal, as shown by the similarity in D values and D versus temperature curves for liquid inactivation in culture medium vs. bovine serum. This is in marked contrast to our findings [6] for the flaviviruses Zika virus, bovine viral diarrhea virus and West Nile virus, where dry heating at 56°C was much more effective in the absence compared to the presence of a high organic load.

There have been few reports on heat inactivation of adenovirus. Maheswari et al. [28] evaluated liquid heat inactivation and observed over a 7.5 $\log_{10}$ reduction in titer following 10 min heating at 70°C. This corresponds to a D of ~1.3 min at this temperature. Tuladhar et al. [29] examined liquid heating of Ad5 in the presence of organic load (1% stool) and in culture medium. The D values at 73°C were 0.53 and 0.40 min, respectively [29]. This indicated a minor impact of organic load on heat inactivation, as we found in the present study.

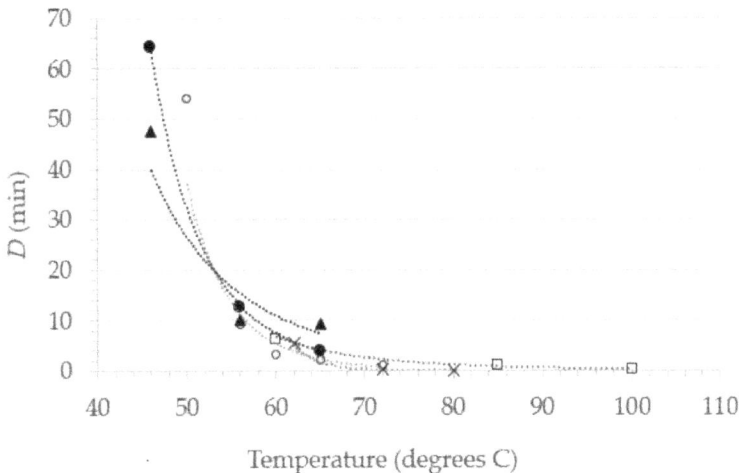

Figure 3. D vs. temperature relationships for heat inactivation of PV-1 in Medium (●) or Serum (▲) liquid matrices; comparison to hepatitis A virus inactivation in culture medium (✕, Ref. [24]) or in homogenates of mussels (O; Ref. [25]) and (□; Ref. [26]).

Comparisons between carrier and liquid heat inactivation for adenoviruses have not been reported. Sauerbrei and Wutzler [9] found Ad5 to be relatively resistant to dry heating. Their data indicate a D value of 67 min at 75°C [9]. This is very discrepant from our carrier results for Ad5. The reason is not clear, although the time kinetics for inactivation were not studied in detail in the previous study (time points included 60 and 120 min only). In our study, clear differences between liquid heating and dry (carrier) heating were observed primarily at 46°C, as the time kinetics were relatively similar for the higher temperatures evaluated.

Questions regarding the impact of organic load and carrier versus liquid heating on the efficacy of thermal inactivation of enteroviruses spread by the fecal-oral route are relevant in achieving adequate disinfection of surfaces in healthcare settings where such viruses might be present in organic-containing physiological substrates (blood, sputum, feces, etc.). It has been shown that transfer of infectious virus from contaminated fomites to humans can result in acquisition of disease [30, 31]. It is important therefore to collect information on the utility of different inactivation approaches, whether these are chemical or physical that might be used to disinfect contaminated fomites. Our results with two enteroviruses from different nonenveloped families suggest that the efficacy of heat inactivation assessed in a liquid versus carrier test format varies according to the virus under evaluation. If extent of heat inactivation is dependent more on the protein composition of the virus than the presence or absence of a lipid envelope, perhaps the differences observed for these two enteroviruses are not unexpected. The variability observed, even among these two nonenveloped viruses, suggests that extrapolation of carrier versus liquid inactivation efficacy should not be made across virus families. As a result, we are now conducting similar studies with a wider range of viruses to more fully characterize the requirements for heat inactivation under these varied conditions.

5. Our interpretation of heat inactivation data

Historically, the relationship between D and temperature has been displayed in plots of $\log_{10} D$ versus temperature (e.g., **Figure 4**). The slope of the (typically) linear relationship thus generated is equivalent to $-1/z$. The z value so obtained can then be used to predict D values at other (nonmeasured) temperatures, using the rather cumbersome formula shown in Eq. (4):

$$\log_{10} D_{predicted} = \log_{10} D_{ref} - \frac{T_{predicted} - T_{ref}}{z} \qquad (4)$$

where $T_{predicted}$ is the temperature at which D is to be predicted and T_{ref} is the temperature at which D_{ref} was actually measured [32]. On the other hand, the plotting of D versus temperature is much more straightforward and intuitive and is occasionally seen in the inactivation literature (e.g., [29]).

The utility of the plot of D versus temperature is greatly enhanced when the power function line fit is added to the plots, as has been done in **Figures 1–3**. The resulting fit lines may be viewed as surfaces along which any temperature and D-value pair is associated with 1 $\log_{10}$ inactivation. The extrapolation of D to nonempirical temperatures that requires some effort using the z values therefore becomes quite easy and straightforward using the D vs. temperature power curve plots.

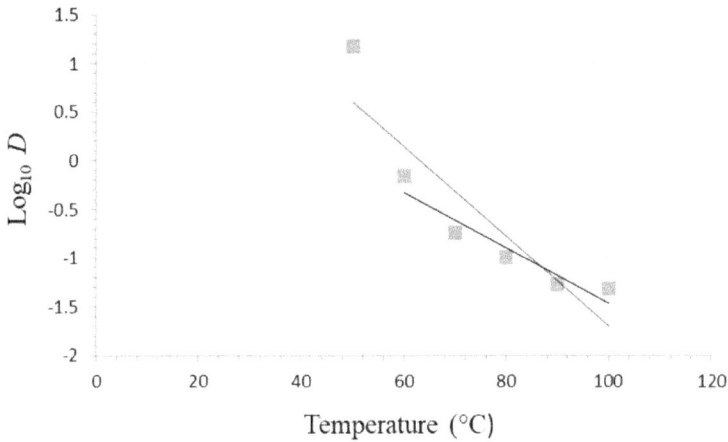

Figure 4. A plot of $\log_{10}D$ vs. temperature for heat inactivation of the OPN strain of the Picornavirus foot and mouth disease virus (Figure from [18], data are from reference [33]).

The nonlinear relationship displayed in the D versus temperature plot (**Figures 1–3**), with the steep portion of the curve at relatively lower temperatures followed by a flattening out at higher temperatures, is more informative also from a mechanism of inactivation point of view than the $\log_{10} D$ versus temperature plot. If heat inactivation is attributed to capsid opening followed by nuclease destruction of genomic material [2, 3], then the steep portion of the curve may represent reaching a threshold temperature required for capsid opening. Once this threshold temperature has been reached, relatively small incremental increases in temperature result in dramatic decreases in the time required for 1 $\log_{10}$ inactivation. Differences between carrier and liquid heat inactivation observed at the lower end of the D versus temperature plot might then correspond to differences in extent or kinetics of heat exchange or other factors to be described below.

There are frequent errors associated with calculation of D values and our own results are not immune to this, as we acknowledged in the methods section earlier. Some might argue that the concept behind the D value for heat inactivation is not always correct. The implication behind D values is that heat inactivation at a given temperature is first order with respect to time, such that a constant $\log_{10}$ inactivation occurs within a given unit of time. In reality, the time frames over which linear behavior is observed experimentally are very short at high temperatures and are limited by the titers of the virus stocks being inactivated. At lower temperatures, extended contact times are required to obtain several $\log_{10}$ of inactivation, so again the determinations of D values can be challenging. In addition, there is always a degree of error associated with the measurement of virus titers before and after heat treatment. D values at three or more different temperatures are required for calculation of power function coefficients and for determining z values, so thoroughly characterizing heat inactivation efficacy in this manner is a rather complicated endeavor.

In general, experimental error associated with calculation of D values translates to poorer linear line fits (i.e., lower coefficients of determination or R^2 values) in the $\log_{10}D$ versus temperature curves. Since the D versus temperature relationship is merely a transformation of the $\log_{10}D$ versus temperature relationship, we have routinely noted that deviations from linearity for the $\log_{10}D$ versus temperature plots (such as those shown in **Figure 4**) are associated with poorer power function fits for the D versus temperature curves generated from the same inactivation results. In **Figure 4**, the R^2 value for the line fit to all six points is 0.82, while the R^2 value for the line fit only to the higher five points is 0.90. The corresponding R^2 values for the power function fits are 0.89 (for all six points) and 0.94 (for the highest five points). The two constants (*a* and *b*) from the power function equation (Eq. (2)) are derived from the *y*-intercept and slope, respectively, from the linear line equation (Eq. (1)) of the corresponding $\log_{10}D$ versus temperature plots.

In sum, regardless of the method used for the analysis of heat inactivation results, it is the D value itself that is the source of most error. However, the conclusions made above regarding efficacy of heat inactivation applied to viruses in solution versus viruses dried on carriers, or the impact of organic load on heat inactivation, can be made directly by evaluation of the raw inactivation data itself. Therefore, the difficulties associated with the appropriateness or accuracy of the D value concept do not detract from our overall conclusions regarding heat inactivation of these two enteroviruses.

6. Executive summary

- Virus inactivation by chemical and physical means may be evaluated either in liquid studies or in carrier studies.

- Liquid inactivation studies are relevant to a barrier or clearance process intended to reduce the viral titer of a solution, while carrier inactivation studies are relevant for surface disinfection approaches.

- A greater volume of virus inactivation data exists in the literature for liquid, relative to carrier, inactivation. Very few studies have compared liquid and carrier inactivation in a side-by-side design.

- Prevailing opinion has been that viruses are less susceptible to heat inactivation in the carrier format relative to the liquid format. Our studies have not confirmed this.

- We found that PV-1 was much more susceptible to inactivation at 46°C on carriers than in liquids, while the susceptibility to inactivation at 65°C was similar for both test formats.

- We found that Ad5 was only slightly more susceptible to inactivation at 46°C on carriers than in liquids, while the susceptibility to 65°C was similar for both test formats.

- Regardless of study format (liquid or carrier) complete inactivation of PV-1 occurred within 20 min at 65°C, while 1 h was required at this temperature to completely inactivate Ad5.

- The presence or absence of increased organic load in the liquid inactivation matrix did not impact heat inactivation efficacy for either PV-1 or Ad5.

- The decimal reduction value (*D*) versus temperature relationship is described well by a power function line fit and the resulting line fit equation may be used in a straightforward manner to extrapolate $\log_{10}$ reduction in virus titer from empirically tested temperatures to other temperatures of interest.

7. Future perspectives

Inactivation studies performed in solutions have been useful in providing comparative efficacy data for different physical and chemical inactivation approaches targeting a given virus or for comparing the intra- and inter-family susceptibilities of different viruses to a given inactivation approach. The current rankings of viruses in terms of susceptibilities to such approaches (e.g., [34, 35]) have largely been derived from liquid inactivation studies. The results of liquid inactivation studies should not be extrapolated to inactivation of viruses on surfaces, however. This is because differences in presentation of the virus to the active, in diffusion of the active through the liquid or virus film (for chemical approaches) or in penetrability of radiation to the viruses or in kinetics of heat exchange (for physical approaches), almost certainly exist. Such differences may favor inactivation in one or the other of the liquid or carrier formats. Generalizations on the relative sensitivities of viruses to inactivation on carriers versus in liquids should not be made in the absence of data. Side-by-side carrier and liquid inactivation studies such as the ones described in this chapter are needed to elucidate the possible differences in efficacy for the various chemical and physical inactivation approaches. This aspect of the inactivation literature is in its infancy, but with time it is expected that the database will continue to grow.

As more sophisticated thinking about the relationship between our environmental microbiome and public health has been evolving, arguments have been made that the current approach to surface disinfection should change. In other words, there is a viewpoint that advocates replacement of the current "sterilization approach' with the use of "smart" antimicrobial agents that target the pathogens while sparing the nonpathogenic population [36]. Heat is, in some regards, capable of serving as a targeted inactivation approach. This is due to the rather striking differences in heat inactivation sensitivity of various viruses or, indeed, various microorganisms in general. At least for the moment though, and especially where viruses are concerned, it would appear that our current "sterilization" approach to heat inactivation will prevail, as we are not overly concerned about the possibility of nonpathogenic viruses competing with pathogenic ones.

Author details

S. Steve Zhou[1]*, Cameron Wilde[1], Zheng Chen[1], Tanya Kapes[1], Jennifer Purgill[1], Raymond Nims[2] and Donna Suchmann[1]

*Address all correspondence to: steve.zhou@microbac.com

1 Microbac Laboratories, Sterling, VA, USA

2 RMC Pharmaceutical Solutions, Inc., Longmont, CO, USA

References

[1]   Nims RW, Plavsic M. Intra-family and inter-family comparisons for viral susceptibility to heat inactivation. Journal of Microbial and Biochemical Technology. 2013;**5**:136-141

[2]   Boschetti N, Wyss K, Mischler A, Hostettler T, Kemph C. Stability of minute virus of mice against temperature and sodium hydroxide. Biologicals. 2003;**31**:181-185

[3]   Nims RW, Zhou SS. Intra-family differences in efficacy of inactivation of small, non-enveloped viruses. Biologicals. 2016;**44**:456-462

[4]   Blümel J, Schmidt I, Willkommen H, Löwer J. Inactivation of parvovirus B19 during pasteurization of human serum albumin. Transfusion. 2002;**42**:1011-1018

[5]   Doerrbecker J, Friesland M, Ciesek S, Erichsen TJ, Mateu-Gelabert P, Steinmann J, Steinmann J, Pietschmann T, Steinmann E. Inactivation and survival of hepatitis C virus on inanimate surfaces. Journal of Infectious Diseases. 2011;**204**:1830-1838

[6]   Wilde C, Chen Z, Kapes T, Chiossone C, Lukula S, Suchmann D, Nims R, Zhou SS. Inactivation and disinfection of Zika virus on a nonporous surface. Journal of Microbial and Biochemical Technology. 2016;**8**:422-427

[7]   McDevitt J, Rudnick S, First M, Spengler J. Role of absolute humidity in the inactivation of influenza viruses on stainless steel surfaces at elevated temperatures. Applied and Environmental Microbiology. 2010;**76**:3943-3947

[8]   Thomas PR, Karriker LA, Ramirez A, Zhang J, Ellingson JS, Crawford KK, Bates JL, Hammen KJ, Holtkamp DJ. Evaluation of time and temperature sufficient to inactivate porcine epidemic diarrhea virus in swine feces on metal surfaces. The Journal of Swine Health & Production. 2015;**23**:84-90

[9]   Sauerbrei A, Wutzler P. Testing thermal resistance of viruses. Archives of Virology. 2009;**154**:115-119

[10] Dekker A. Inactivation of foot-and-mouth disease virus by heat, formaldehyde, ethylene oxide and Υ-irradiation. The Veterinary Record. 1998;**143**:168-169

[11] Bräuninger S, Peters S, Borchers U, Kao M. Further studies on thermal resistance of bovine parvovirus against moist and dry heat. International Journal of Hygiene and Environmental Health. 2000;**203**:71-75

[12] von Rheinbaben F, Wolff MH. Handbuch der viruswirksamen Desinfektion. Berlin: Springer; 2002. pp. 1-499

[13] Howard RS. Poliomyelitis. In: Hilton-Jones D, Turner MR, editors. Oxford Textbook of Neuromuscular Disorders. Oxford: Oxford University Press; 2014. pp. 51-60

[14] Wood DJ. Adenovirus gastroenteritis. British Medical Journal. 1988;**296**:229-230

[15] ASTM E1053. Test method to assess virucidal activity of chemicals intended for disinfection of inanimate, nonporous environmental surfaces. West Conshohocken, PA: ASTM International; 2011

[16] ASTM E1052. Standard test method to assess the activity of microbicides against viruses in suspension. West Conshohocken, PA: ASTM International; 2011

[17] Finney DJ. Statistical Methods in Biological Assay. 2nd ed. London: Griffen; 1964

[18] Nims R, Plavsic M. A proposed modeling approach for comparing the heat inactivation susceptibility of viruses. Bioprocessing Journal. 2013;**12**(2):25-35

[19] Kramer A, Schwebke I, Kampf G. How long do nosocomial pathogens persist on inanimate surfaces? A systematic review. BMC Infectious Diseases. 2006;**6**:130. DOI: 10.1186/1471-2334-6-130

[20] Boone SA, Gerba CP. Significance of fomites in the spread of respiratory and enteric viral disease. Applied and Environmental Microbiology. 2007;**73**:1687-1696

[21] Sattar SA, Springthorpe VS, Karim YK, Loro P. Chemical disinfection of non-porous inanimate surfaces experimentally contaminated with four human pathogenic viruses. Epidemiology and Infection. 1989;**102**:493-505

[22] Sattar SA, Springthorpe VS, Adegbunrin O, Abu Zafer A, Busa M. A disc-based quantitative carrier test method to assess the virucidal activity of chemical germicides. The Journal of Virological Methods. 2003;**112**:3-12

[23] Rabenau HF, Steinmann J, Rapp I, Schwebke I, Eggers M. Evaluation of a virucidal quantitative carrier test for surface disinfectants. PLoS One. 2014;**9**:e86128. DOI: 10:1371/journal.pone.0086128

[24] Araud E, DiCaprio E, Ma Y, Lou F, Gao Y, Kingsley D, Hughes JH, Li J. Thermal inactivation of enteric viruses and bioaccumulation of enteric foodborne viruses in live oysters (*Crassostrea virginica*). Applied and Environmental Microbiology. 2016;**82**:2086-2099

[25] Bozkurt H, D'Souza DH, Davidson PM. Determination of thermal inactivation kinetics of hepatitis a virus in blue mussel (*Mytilus edulis*) homogenate. Applied and Environmental Microbiology. 2014;**83**:3191-3197

[26] Park SY, Ha S-D. Thermal inactivation of hepatitis a in suspension and in dried mussels (*Mytilus edulis*). International Journal of Food Science and Technology. 2014;**50**:717-722

[27] Bozkurt H, D'Souza DH, Davidson PM. Thermal inactivation of foodborne enteric viruses and their viral surrogates in foods. Journal of Food Protection. 2015;**78**:1597-1617

[28] Maheshwari G, Jannat R, McCormick L, Hsu D. Thermal inactivation of adenovirus type 5. The Journal of Virological Methods. 2004;**118**:141-146

[29] Tuladhar E, Bouwknegt M, Zwietering MH, Koopmans M, Duizer E. Thermal stability of structurally different viruses with proven or potential relevance to food safety. Journal of Applied Microbiology. 2012;**112**:1050-1057

[30] Ward RL, Bernstein DI, Knowlton DR, Sherwood JR, Young EC, Cusack TM, Rubino JR, Schiff GM. Prevention of surface-to-human transmission of rotaviruses by treatment with disinfectant spray. Journal of Clinical Microbiology. 1991;**29**:1991-1996

[31] Oristo S, Rönnqvist M, Aho M, Sovijärva A, Hannila-Handelberg T, Hörman A, Nikkari S, Kinnunen PM, Maunula L. Contamination by norovirus and adenovirus on environmental surfaces and in hands of conscripts in two Finnish garrisons. Food and Environmental Virology. 2017;9:62-71

[32] van Asselt ED, Zwietering MH. A systematic approach to determine global thermal pathogen inactivation parameters for various food pathogens. International Journal of Food Microbiology 2006;107:73-82

[33] Kamolsiripichaiporn S, Subharat S, Udon R, Thongtha P, Nuanualsuwan S. Thermal inactivation of foot-and-mouth disease viruses in suspension. Applied and Environmental Microbiology. 2007;73:7177-7184

[34] United States Pharmacopeia. <1050.1> Design, evaluation and characterization of viral clearance procedures The United States Pharmacopeial Convention, Inc.

[35] International Conference on Harmonisation (ICH). Q5A (R1) Viral safety evaluation of biotechnology products derived from cell lines of human or animal origin. 1997. http://www.ich.org/fileadmin/Public_Web_Site/ICH_Products/Guidelines/Quality/Q5A_R1/Step4/Q5A_R1__Guideline.pdf

[36] Scott EA, Bruning E, Ijaz MK. Targeted decontamination of environmental surfaces in everyday settings. In: Mc Donnell G, Hansen J, editors. Block's Disinfection, Sterilization and Preservation. 6th ed. Philadelphia: Wolters Kluwer; in press

Chemical Analysis of By-products

Chapter 4

New Trends in Chemical Analysis of Disinfection By-Products

Milton Rosero-Moreano

Additional information is available at the end of the chapter

http://dx.doi.org/10.5772/intechopen.77254

Abstract

The disinfection by-products are special category of emergent pollutants, and their formation is widely known when the organic matter present in the catchment water reaches the disinfection agent in the water treatment plants. These kinds of compounds are close to more than 500 molecules classified in the following main families: halomethanes, haloacetic acids, haloacetonitriles and haloketones. Their adverse effects in the health are widely recognized for international health organisms and normally are in trace levels that promote the development of smart strategies for their analysis in aquatic environments where these compounds are generally not alone. In this way, the microextraction techniques for analysis of emergent contaminants in the environment which are in trace amounts have gained a lot of space because they comply fully with the objectives established in the sample preparation field: reduction in the number of steps, adaptability to field sampling, automation and reduction or total elimination of solvents required for extraction by meeting in one step the main tasks of any sample preparation technique: extraction, clean up and enrichment. There are a lot of possibilities in this field: solid phase microextraction (SPME), liquid phase microextraction (LPME), stir bar sorptive extraction (SBSE) and rotating disk sorptive extraction (RDSE).

Keywords: microextraction, disinfection by-products, halomethanes, haloacetic acids, water treatment plant, solid phase microextraction, chemical risk

1. Introduction

The sample preparation SP is the most critical step and on it is spent a lot of time in the chemical analysis, in addition herein the people make the higher number of mistakes in the whole procedure, so that in other words the SP is the "neck of bottle" of analytical procedure.

IntechOpen

In special, this step turn off more difficult when the matrices to analyze are foods, complex materials or the target analytes are in trace amounts. Taking into account the above premises and the ideology of green chemistry based on: elimination or reduction of organic solvents, reduction of the steps number in the procedure, integration and automation of sampling and analysis in just one step, by leading to more eco-efficient and productive analytical procedures. That allows to reach the three major challenges on sample preparation: isolation, cleanup and preconcentration with better practices an optimum results [1]. In this way, the solventless microextraction techniques have gained a lot of space because fully comply with the objectives and goals above established. Additionally, they meet in one step the main tasks of any sample preparation technique: extraction, clean up and enrichment.

The disinfection by-products (DBPs) are a special kind of compounds which appear in a trace amounts during the chlorination processes in the water treatment plants (WTP). These low concentrations represent a challenge for analytical chemists. The aqueous matrices are easier to manage than sludge, air or biological fluids because the presence of interferences are low, but some of these compounds are volatile and other are nonvolatile and polar analytes, that drives to take a compromise decision for that in a single run can analyze all these compounds by facilitating the through routine in a laboratory water analysis. In this sense, the microextraction techniques help to reach the low requested detection limits for the preconcentration factor as a special characteristic of these kind of procedures. By the other side, there are the possibilities to eliminate interferences and to use a minimal amount of organic solvents. Taking into account that all this valuable merit figures are possible to do in one step, the automation operation have been reached easily.

2. Chemical formation of disinfection by-products and health implications

The disinfection process in the water treatment plant is a routine practice for microbial control risk due to the presence in raw water of the microbial pathogens. The disinfection agent more widespread is chlorine for its effectiveness, low cost, easier management and high residual effect for assurance protection along to the distribution network.

2.1. The formation reaction of disinfection by-products: natural organic matter (NOM) + Chlorine

Rook in 1974 had established that the disinfection by-products formation is due to reaction between natural organic matter NOM and chlorine [2, 3]. The NOM precedence is basically from leaching tannin compounds from leaves and soil, which have a common structure of polyphenol rings (resorcinol-type molecules) [4, 5]. The primary disinfection by-products results from breakage under chlorine influence of polyphenol ring through the next three pathways a, b and c, such as is shown in **Figure 1**.

As shown in **Figure 1**, if the breakage is by pathway *a*, it will form halomethanes, through pathway *b* with insertion of a hydroxide, the haloacetic acids and the pathway *c* will produce haloketones. From these primary DPBs and the reaction with bromine or iodine inclusively

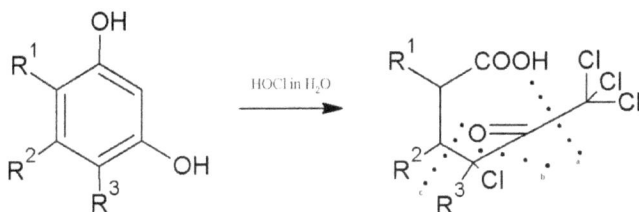

Figure 1. Mechanism of the DBP's formation.

the mixture between alone primary disinfection by-products will occur the emergent or secondary DPBs such as bromohalomethane, iodotrihalomethane, haloacetonitrile, etc. These last inclusively with a higher chemical risk for the health due to higher toxicity in the bromine and iodine atoms [6].

2.2. The pondering risk: microbial versus chemical risk

The chronic risk is associated with cancer's presence due to intake of foods with toxic chemical compounds, this is the case of DBPs in the drinking water, and their effects normally are developed in advanced ages of human being but the acute risk related with microbial infection due to presence of the microbial pathogens show their consequences immediately and their effects can be mortally. The drinking water is a good scenery for pondering the effects and consequences of damage between the chemical associated with presence of DBPs and for the other side with microbial issues due to bacteria diseases related with bacterial contamination. The dosage application of disinfectant in the drinking water is in all development countries (emergent countries) a measure to prevent the microbial risk due to its accelerated development and tragic consequences but simultaneously formation of chemical compounds and many evidences of cancer formation has been done.

The issue in the disinfection proposals in the water treatment plants is the key for control of both risks, that means to find the ideal chlorine dosage for avoiding and diminishing the microbial problem and for other way to control the formation of DBPs in big amounts that represents a severe risk to the drinking water servers [7–9].

2.3. The disinfection by-products and regulations

The disinfection by-products DBPs are cataloged as emergent contaminants, [10] due to its recognized effects to the health and that its formation is frequently in the WTP and the exposition is high and direct by the culture of consumption of drinking water during all day without a forbidden recommendation of the authorities.

Table 1 shows the different normatives and rules with respect to control and prevention directives of DBPs under the guidance of health and technical institutions with wide knowledge in the target issue.

The most known DPBs are the trihalomethanes THMs, then the haloacetic acids HAA, allows in the importance and recognition the HAN haloacetonitrile. Nowadays, the emergent DBPs have become important in the emergent DBPs due to lower and trace amounts, meanwhile more severe and toxic health effects, such as bromohalomethanes and iodohalomethanes.

Item	Organization	DBPs	Value $\mu g\ L^{-1}$	IARC Health Categories*	Ref.
1	World Health Organization (WHO) $\frac{[CH\,Cl_3]}{200} + \frac{[CH\,Cl_2\,Br]}{60} + \frac{[CH\,Cl\,Br_2]}{100} + \frac{[CH\,Br_3]}{100} = 1$	Chloroform	200	Group 2B	[11, 14, 22]
		Bromodichloromethane	60	Group 2B	
		Dibromochloromethane	100	Group 3	
		Bromoform	100	Group 3	
		Dichloroacetic acid	50	Group 2B	
		Trichloroacetic acid	100	Group 3	
		Dichloroacetonitrile	90	Group 3	
		Dibromoacetonitrile	100	Group 2B	
		Trichloroacetonitrile	1	Group 3	
2	Environmental Protection Agency (EPA)	Chloroform	30	Group 2B	[12, 22]
		TTHMs	80	Group 3	
		Haloacetic acids	60	Group 2B	
3	European Union (EU)	Total trihalomethanes	100	Group 3	[13, 22]
4	South Korean Regulation	Total trihalomethanes	100	Group 3	[47]
		Haloacetic acids	100	Group 2B	
		Dichloroacetonitrile	90	Group 3	
		Dibromoacetonitrile	100	Group 2B	
		Trichloroacetonitrile	4	Group 3	
5	Australian Regulatory Limits	Trihalomethanes	250	Group 3	[43]
6	Colombian Regulation	Trihalomethanes	200	Group 3	[23]

*Group 1: the agent is carcinogenic to humans; Group 2A: the agent is probably carcinogenic to humans; Group 2B: the agent is possibly carcinogenic to humans; Group 3: the agent is not classifiable as to its carcinogenicity to humans; Group 4: the agent is probably not carcinogenic to humans [14].

Table 1. Rules, guides and regulation normatives to prevent and control of DBPs for drinking water ($\mu g\ L^{-1}$).

2.4. The health implications and evidences WHO and IARC

The epidemiological and toxicological evidences of cancer by drinking water with contents higher that mentioned guidelines in **Table 1** have been demonstrated in numerous cases, this is correlated with consumer's frequency and anatomical and physiological conditions of town server [7, 8, 11–14]. The difference among the several DBPs fill down in to the carcinogenic categories, there being two well defined kinds: possible and probable carcinogenic agent in dependence of the number of incidence and prevalence cases. In **Table 1**, this remarkable issue is shown and explained for each one DBPs.

2.5. The alternative disinfectants

Taking into account the health implications of DBP's present in the drinking water as result of the reaction between NOM and chlorine in the WTP but with the imperious necessity by controlling the action of microbial pathogens in the raw water due to uncontrolled wastewater discharges into the catchment water, has been raised the use of other alternative disinfectants with the same or better properties than chlorine or chloride derivatives: effectiveness, low cost, easy management and big residual effect. Among candidates can be mentioned are as follows: ozone, hydrogen peroxide, UV-light, potassium permanganate, peroxyacetic acid,and so on [15].

Ozone: the ozone O_3 has a good effectiveness, high cost, technical management and low residual effect. It is properly used in the industrial deals.

Hydrogen peroxide: The hydrogen peroxide H_2O_2 has a medium effectiveness, low cost, technical management and low residual effect. Its use is widespread for catalytic experiments as ·OH promoter in Fenton or pseudo Fenton reactions.

UV-light: This physical source of disinfectant has high effectiveness, high cost, technical management and low residual effect. This is properly for condominial and individual solutions of supplier drinking water. Its drawbacks with the cost can diminish in permanent solar offer places.

Potassium permanganate: The $KMnO_4$ is a strong oxidant close to 1.1 eV. It has good effectiveness, low cost, technical management and high residual effect but to the moment are unknown its by-products formation, letting a strong flavor and taste of final drinking water and can increase the network damage due to its strong oxidation capacity.

Peroxyacetic acid: $C_2H_4O_3$ is an emergent sanitizer in the market for agricultural, medical environments, water and wastewater industry, food processing, beverage and pharmaceutical industries. It has good effectiveness, low cost, easy management and medium residual effects due to depletion into its precursors: hydrogen peroxide and acetic acid promotes by heat and bad storage and obviously letting low admissible characteristic flavor and taste to the drinking water [15].

As can inference from the mentioned alternatives disinfectants, we are so far to find soon a replacement to the chlorine.

2.6. The disinfection: Pondering between microbial and chemical risks

Some researchers like Craun [7–9] have established a basic model to pondering the weight and evolution of both risks associated and in interdependence with the chlorine dosage practice in the WTP (see **Figure 2**).

As shown in **Figure 2**, and with strict dependence of formation reaction of DBPs, there are two ways for controlling in the just measures both risks: to have good quality raw water (that means low precursors amounts and microbes) and to do a rationalize chlorine dosage practice.

2.7. Classification of disinfection by-products

There are at least 500 chemical compounds catalogued as disinfection by-products [16], which are classified in four great families:

- Halomethanes
- Haloacetic acids
- Haloketones
- Haloacetonitriles

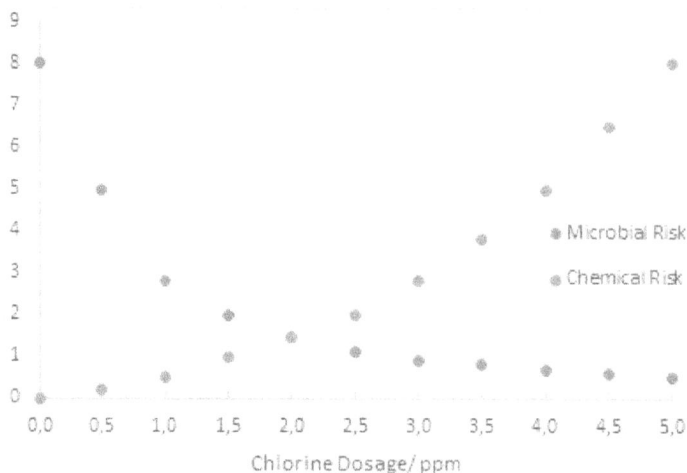

Figure 2. Pondering the microbial and chemical risk in the disinfection practice with chlorine.

These compounds are also catalogued as emergent contaminants due to widespread use or formation and uncontrolled measures by sanitary authorities.

In **Table 2**, it is shown the DBPs classification containing the most cited molecules, their chemical formula and some references about found reported cases.

2.8. Routinely chemical analysis of DBPs

Due to their physicochemical condition, the most disinfection by-products are volatile and non or low polar compounds. In this sense, the proper chemical way for their analysis is the gas chromatography (GC) coupled with electron capture detection (ECD) for the presence in the molecule of electronegative atoms (halogens) or MS. In special for haloacetic acids due to their low vapor pressure and to be polar molecules is preferable the liquid chromatography by UV-detection or to derivatize to their methylesther derivatives (volatile and nonpolar compounds) with methanol under acidic conditions and catalize by anhydride chloroacetic, by doing possible their analysis by GC.

2.8.1. Liquid: liquid extraction

The USEPA method 502 established the liquid–liquid extraction (LLE) as official method for their analysis based on their physicochemical properties (**Table 2**). To 20 mL of aqueous sample to be add 5 mL of hexane, pentane or MtBE as extraction organic solvent into a 50 mL separation funnel, then the mixture is degasified by opening the key's funnel with the separation funnel slightly inclined, this operation is done by five times and then returns to initial and vertical position. Then let be the funnel in vertical position overnight to warranty the complete separation of both phases organic and aqueous, passed this time to recover the

Family	Compound	Chemical Formula	Molar mass g mol^{-1}	CAS	B.p. °C	Log P	Ref.
Halomethanes	Chloroform	CHCl$_3$	119.37	67-66-3	61.2	1.83	[41]
	Dibromochloro methane	CHBr$_2$Cl	208.28	124-48-1	119	2.13	[41]
	Bromodichloro methane	CHCl$_2$Br	163.82	75-27-4	90	1.98	
	Bromoform	CHBr$_3$	252.731	75-25-2	149.1	2.28	
Haloacetic Acids	Monochloroacetic acid (MCA)	C$_2$H$_3$ClO$_2$	94.49	79-11-8	189.3	0.31	[48]
	Bromochloroacetic acid (BCA)	C$_2$H$_2$Cl$_2$O$_2$	128.94	79-43-6	194	1.06	
	Dichloroacetic acid (DCA)	C$_2$HCl$_3$O$_2$	163.38	76-03-9	196	1.53	
	Trichloroacetic acid (TCA)	C$_2$H$_3$BrO$_2$	138.948	79-08-3	208	0.50	
	Monobromoacetic acid (MBA)	C$_2$H$_2$Br$_2$O$_2$	217.844	631-64-1	128	0.70	
	Dibromoacetic acid (DBA)	C$_2$HBr$_3$O$_2$	296.74	N/A	245	1.98	
	Tribromoacetic acid (TBA)	C$_2$H$_2$BrClO$_2$	173.39	5589-96-8	210	0.79	
	Dichlorobromoacetic acid (DCBA)	C$_2$HBrCl$_2$O$_2$	207.83	71133-14-7	N/A	1.68	
	Dibromochloroacetic acid (DBCA)	C$_2$HBr$_2$ClO$_2$	252.29	5278-95-5	N/A	1.83	
Haloketones	1,1-dichloropropanone (1,1-DCP)	C$_3$H$_4$Cl$_2$O	126.96	513-88-2	118	1.39	[22, 48]
	1,3-dichloropropanone (1,3-DCP)	C$_3$H$_4$Cl$_2$O	126.96	534-07-6	173	1.18	
	1,1,1-trichloropropanone (1,1,1-TCP)	C$_3$H$_3$Cl$_3$O	161.41	918-00-3	134	1.86	
Haloacetonitrile	Monochloroacetonitrile (MCAN)	C$_2$H$_2$ClN	75.5	107-14-2	124	0.37	[47]
	Monobromoacetonitrile (MBAN)	C$_2$H$_2$BrN	119.949	590-17-0	60	0.56	[48]
	Dibromoacetonitrile (DBAN)	C$_2$HBr$_2$N	198.845	3252-43-5	67	0.68	
	Dichloroacetonitrile (DCAN)	C$_2$HCl$_2$N	109.94	3018-12-0	110	1.12	
	Trichloroacetonitrile (TCAN)	C$_2$Cl$_3$N	144.38	545-06-2	83	1.59	
	Bromochloroacetonitrile (BCAN)	C$_2$HBrClN	154.39	83463-62-1		0.77	

CAS: Chemical Abstracts Service; B.p: Boiling point.

Table 2. Disinfection by-products classification and physicochemical properties.

organic extract in the overhead (less dense phase) by releasing the aqueous phase, opening the key's funnel and exactly closing when in the funnel there have been just the organic phase, from this phase to take and direct inject into chromatograph equipped with electron capture detection ECD. The yield of this method is calculated in the equation [1]

$$[S]_1 = \frac{[S]_0 V_1}{V_1 + V_2 D} = [S]_0 \left(\frac{1}{1 + D \frac{V_2}{V_1}} \right)$$

(1)

where

$[S]_1$ = Concentration of solute in the phase 1

$[S]_0$ = Initial concentration of solute

V_1 = Aqueous volume phase

V_2 = Organic volume phase

D = Distribution relation

This operation is possible to do n times reaching better results, because in an exhaustive method, in dependence on the next equation [2]

$$[S]_1 = [S]_0 \left(\frac{1}{1+D\frac{V_2}{V_1}} \right)^n \tag{2}$$

2.8.2. Solid phase extraction SPE

This procedure is properly for concentration and cleanup method for nonvolatile compounds [17]. The cartridges available for extraction are SDB, NH_2, C18, C8, HLB, SAX and SCX sorbents. The whole SPE procedure includes four steps: conditioning, loading, wash and elution. It has been used for solid-phase extraction of 35 DBPs with analysis by GC-ECD and GC–MS [18, 19] (**Figure 3**).

2.8.3. Head space extraction HSE

Due the volatility of the major DPBs one very affordable technique for their analysis is the head space extraction, there are in the market two automatized possibilities: with transference line [20–22], and high volume syringe [23, 24]. In both cases, the stirring and heating are promoted by the same equipment, two of the most important and critical variables in the extraction process. In addition and with the similarity concept from Schdmidt's group has come the device coined in tube extraction (ITEX), in this case the high volume syringe are coated with specific sorbent material with big affinity for the target analytes [25].

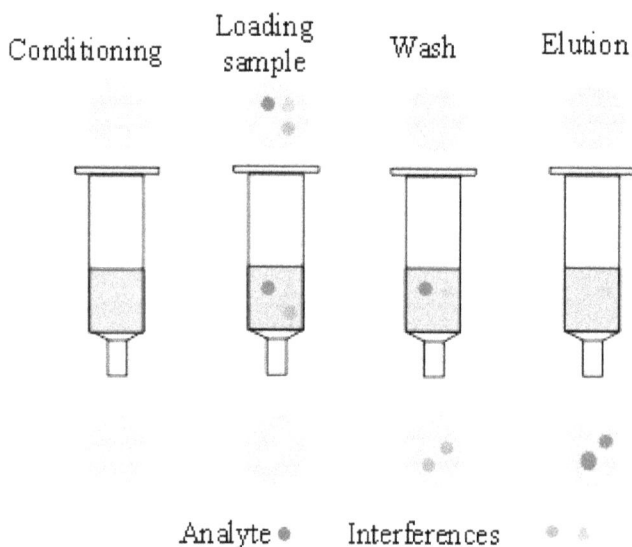

Figure 3. Steps of solid phase extraction SPE.

2.9. New trends in chemical analysis of DBPs

Based on the green chemistry ideology, the new trends in chemical analysis of DBPs advice to lead the sample preparation in route of miniaturization, automation and lower solvent amounts. The first attempts to meet these criteria have been done by Pawliszyn et al. (1989) with the solid phase microextraction (SPME) development [26]. Also, Jeannot [27] in 1997 did miniaturize the liquid–liquid extraction in the form of single drop microextraction (SDME). Then, simultaneously from different origins and countries were developed in 1999: the stir bar sorption extraction (SBSE) and the liquid phase microextraction with hollow fiber (HF-LPME) by Sandra [28] and Pederssen [29], respectively. In 2009, Richter [30] has discovered the rotating disk sorption extraction (RDSE). Thus, in the last three decades smart devices have been invented giving compliment to the goals of the new trends in chemical analysis.

The thermodynamic principles that rules the distribution of analyte from aqueous phase (1) to organic phase (2) are summarized in the next three equations.

$$K = \frac{a_{S_1}}{a_{S_1}} = \frac{[S]_2}{[S]_1} \tag{3}$$

$$R = \frac{K V_2}{K V_2 + V_2} \tag{4}$$

$$EF = \frac{V_1 R}{100 V_2} \tag{5}$$

where

K = distribution or partition constant

$aS_1 = [S]_1$ = Activity or concentration of analyte in aqueous phase

$aS_2 = [S]_2$ = Activity or concentration of analyte in organic phase

V_1 = Volume aqueous phase

V_2 = Volume organic phase

R = Recovery

EF = Enrichment factor

The next extraction techniques to study are equilibrium processes, that means their distribution constants are on strong dependence of temperature, time, ionic force and stirring speed.

2.9.1. Solid phase microextraction SPME

This device consists of a sorbent polymer coating over thin stainless steel wire. It is a robustness, selectivity and powerful technique for volatile compounds, in special for DBPs compounds. There are two working modes: in headspace HS and direct immersion DI. For nonvolatile analytes is possible to lead the derivatization reaction in fiber or out fiber (**Figure 4**).

There are a wide range of polarities of sorbents polymer coatings from nonpolar until polar moieties, allowing a great spectrum of affinities by polarity for extraction of several kinds of molecules, for example, polydimethylsiloxane PDMS, polydivinylbenzene DVB, carboxen [26], and nowadays has been gone gain a lot of terrain, the greener sorbents such as modified clays, cork, agarose, chitosan, magnetite, nanoparticles or nanotubes [31].

2.9.2. Liquid phase microextraction LPME

It is the miniaturization of liquid–liquid extraction (LLE). The basic principle is the distribution or partition of the analyte between aqueous phase and organic phase. The amount of organic phase used is micro amounts from 5 until 30 µL.

2.9.2.1. LPME with protected membrane

In this specific technique, the solvent is supported by a porous polymer membrane. The HF is made in hydrophobic polypropylene (300 µm internal diameter ID; 1.2 mm wall thickness, and 0.2 µm pore size), and act as a filter due to its microporous constitution less than 0.2 µm size pore (**Figure 5**).

2.9.2.1.1. HF-LPME two phases HF-2-LPME

With porous membrane (hollow fiber) used as support for the extractant solvent, there are two specific working modes: in two and three phases. In two mode, the solvent is filled into the hollow fiber (HF) and also dipped into the pores, in other words the solvent is

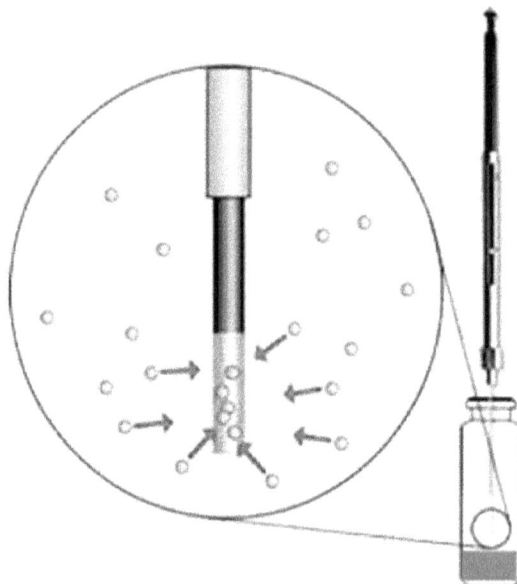

Figure 4. Schematic representation of extraction device by SPME. Source: [26].

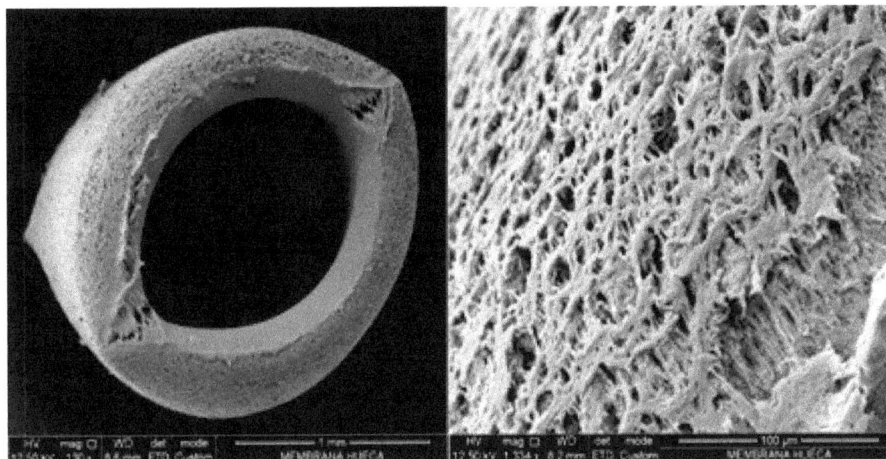

Figure 5. SEM micrographs of HF.

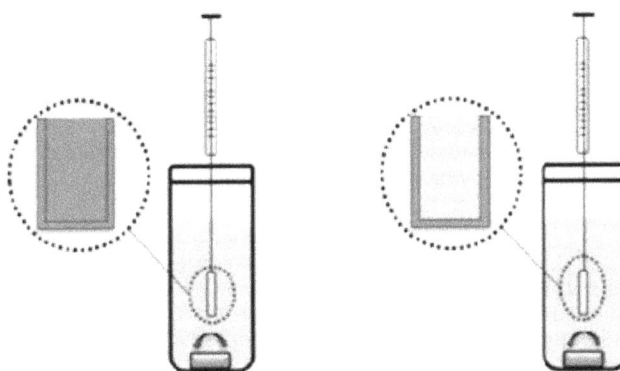

Figure 6. HF liquid phase microextraction modes: Two phases (left); three phases (right). Source: [1].

immobilized in the membrane pore's and filled inside it (**Figure 6**, https://drive.google.com/drive/folders/1dE94Qe_VhY-U3x0909WPIOWpoPtIvVHg). The force that facilitates the transfer mass is the mass gradient.

2.9.2.1.2. HF-LPME three phases HF-3-LPME

As shown in **Figure 6**, the three phases mode implied the immobilization of the organic solvent into the membrane pores, then outsider and insider of HF, both phases are aqueous, normally in this mode is necessary put a pH gradient to enhance the transfer mass. In the donor phase (outsider), the type of pH (acidic o basic aqueous phase) is on dependence of pKa target analyte, in any case herein is important to assure the molecular or neutral form of target molecule to reach higher affinity with organic solvent, and in the insider phase should turn on to ionic form of the analyte in study to avoid the back extraction.

In 2014, we developed the new microextraction technique on hollow fiber liquid phase micro-extraction (HF-LPME) basis [32, 33]. The enhancement consisted in the functionalization of the HF as solvent bar because the stirring promotes a better mass transfer. For this accomplishment, we put a small stainless steel wire into the HF prior to fill it with extracting solvent (preferably 1-octanol). The new approach was coined hollow fiber solvent bar microextraction (HF-SBME) (see **Figure 7** and https://drive.google.com/drive/folders/1dE94Qe_VhY-U3x0909WPIOWpoPtIvVHg), by adding to the early advantages the possibilities to reduce the Nernst's layer diffusion and enhancing the analyte transfer from aqueous to organic phases.

2.9.2.1.3. Electromembrane extraction EME

The EME is a one class of three phase LPME mode, but now the driven force to assure the transfer mass is the external electric force impost under power supply. The electrodes are made in platinum and the electric field necessary is the 10 V. This kind of technique is especially for ionic or ionizable compounds and biological matrices [29].

The extraction process with electromembrane has been carried out with two platinum electrodes 5 cm in length and applying a 10 V potential with power supply Enduro™ 300 V (Labnet International Inc.), through the semipermeable membrane of 50 mm in length (50 μL acceptor medium). Several liquid extractants that served as supporting liquid membrane (SLM) have been analyzed, for example, ionic liquid hexadecyl methylimidazolium hexafluorophosphate $[C_6MIM][PF_6]$, 1-octanol, 2-nitrophenyl octyl ether (NPOE). For analytes with high values of pKa, a conventional reverse electrode arrangement has been used as shown in **Figure 8** and an acidic acceptor medium has been used, while maintaining the analyte ionized at pH near 7 in the donor media.

2.9.2.2. LPME without protected membrane

Is the classic liquid–liquid extraction LLE but using microvolumes of organic solvent. There are two special techniques:

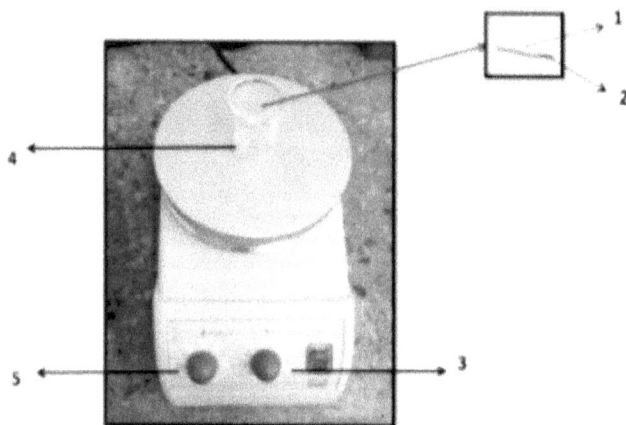

Figure 7. Assembly system of HF-SBME.

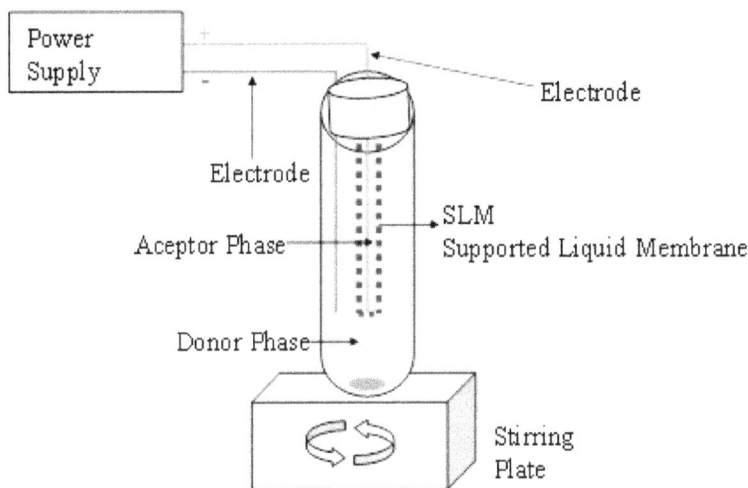

Figure 8. Outline electromembrane EME isolation technique.

2.9.2.2.1. Dispersive liquid–liquid microextraction DLLME

This method involves the dispersion of micro amounts of water-insoluble extraction solvent, normally organic solvent (e.g., chloroform, ionic liquids). This solvent is mixed with 100–500 µL of dispersive agent (methanol normally), followed by the addition of 5 mL of aqueous sample. The whole system has been shaken and further centrifuged (3000 rpm) for 10 min. After centrifugation, a portion of the extracting solvent is concentrated and redissolved in 100 µL of methanol prior to chromatography analysis [34] (**Figure 9**).

2.9.2.2.2. Single drop microextraction SDME

Herein, the miniaturization is concentrated in a single drop (from 1 to 5 µL) of organic solvent which is suspended in a 10 µL Hamilton syringe in a proper holder to assure a stability and avoid the breakout of the drop (**Figure 10**). The organic solvent should be viscous, thermally stable and affordable with the chromatographic system. Also, this extraction mode is possible to do in two formats: direct immersion and headspace.

2.9.3. Stir bar sorption extraction SBSE

The last two microextraction techniques are seemed with the SPME, but these have the advantage to facilitate the mass transfer to the solid sorbent from aqueous sample due to device agitation that allows decrease the stagnant water layer (Nernst's diffusion layer). In special for SBSE, the device has a lot of possibilities to reach the wide sorbent polarities from nonpolar to polar moieties (**Figure 11**).

The research group from Lisbon University headed by Nogueira [38] has been developed a miniaturized SBSE coined as BAµE due to smaller size, giving the possibilities the flotation process with the added issue that has a wider range of sorbent's polarities than original SBSE special for polar target compounds inclusively in one same extraction step has been put two

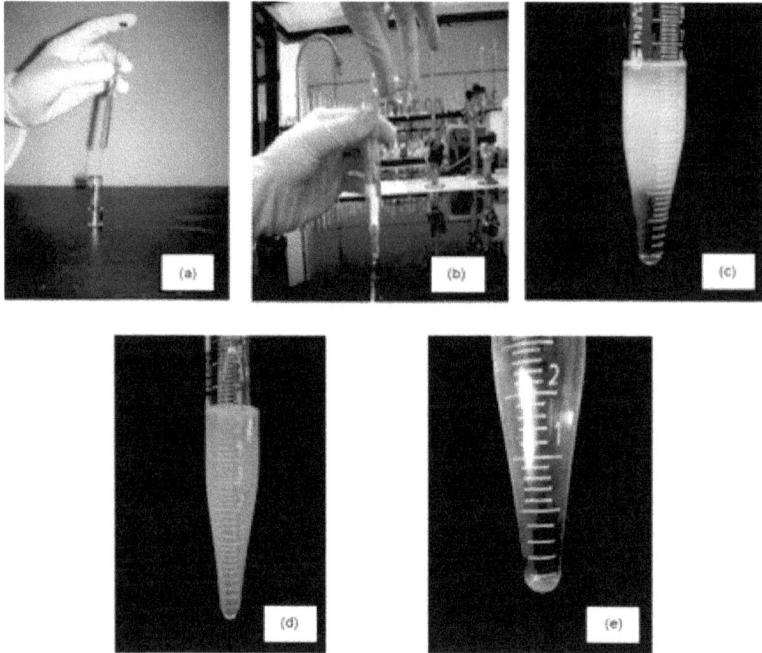

Figure 9. Photography of DLLME. Source: [35].

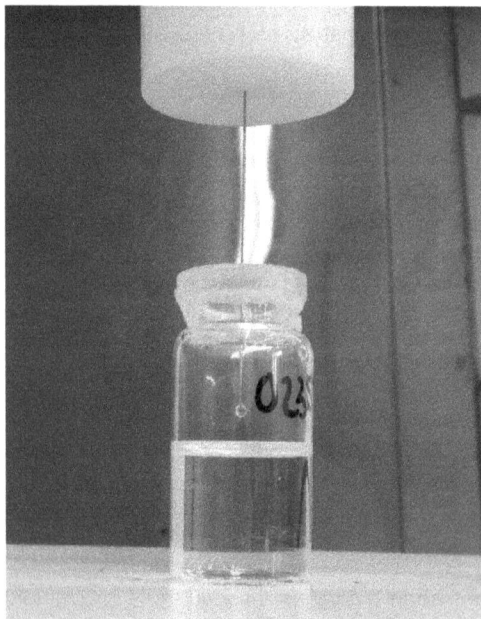

Figure 10. Assembly for single drop microextraction SDME.

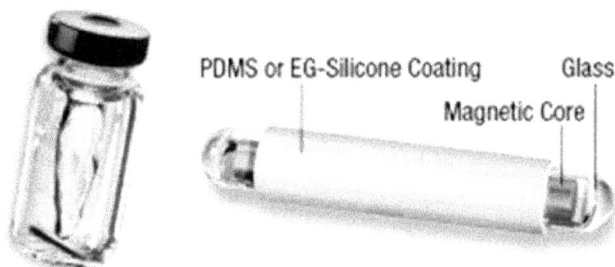

Figure 11. The stir bar sorption extraction (SBSE) representation. Source: [36, 37].

different bars, one of them in flotation and the other one in stirring mode (one bar coated with different sorbent's polarities e.g. PDMS and Carboxen).

2.9.4. Rotating Sorptive disk extraction RDSE

Like that the last microextraction technique, the essential falls in the agitation possibilities, but herein the sorbent phase can be packed or immobilized in the rotating disk made in Teflon with magnet into the body. In both cases, there is no contact between sorbent phase and vial glass of sample, allowing the enlarge shelf life to the extraction sorbent, more tuning abilities respect to the availability of sorbent phases in the market and inclusively faster stirring speed is possible to reach with this device (4000 rpm approx.) and also has the advantage a larger contact surface of the sorbent with the sample allowing satisfactory conditions for extraction and preconcentration of the analytes (**Figure 12**).

2.9.4.1. New sorbent phases and materials

During the last decades, eco-efficiency is acquiring an important position among the typical figures of merit of an analytical methodology [39]. Particularly microextraction techniques have been characterized as a green technology [1] mainly because the use of chemicals is significantly reduced. More recently, the use of eco-sorbents in microextraction techniques have been described such as clays, cork, zeolites, magnetite, biomass, nanotubes, nanoparticules alone or covered with biodegradable material such as agarose, chitosan, polylactic acid PLA, polyhidroxyalcanoate PHA, among others which provides an additional green connotation to this technology [31].

For example, in 2015, we developed a new material by modifying by intercalation way of ionic liquid (IL) based on imidazolium quaternary ammonium salts into the galleries of natural montmorillonite clays (**Figure 13**) has been demonstrated by exhibiting the big possibilities of their use in the extraction and sample preparation field [40]. In this way, the new sorbent MMT-HDMIM-Br developed has been working as a novel solid phase in the rotating disk sorptive extraction with high performance in the PCBs retention, had been exhibited good analytical performance (see **Table 3**).

In 2017, we developed a novel sorptive phase consisting of an ionic liquid intercalated in montmorillonite that has been immobilized onto agarose gel MMT-IL-AF (**Figure 14**). The sorptive phase, a new ecosorbent, has been used in a thin film of 1 mm thickness x 2.5 cm ID

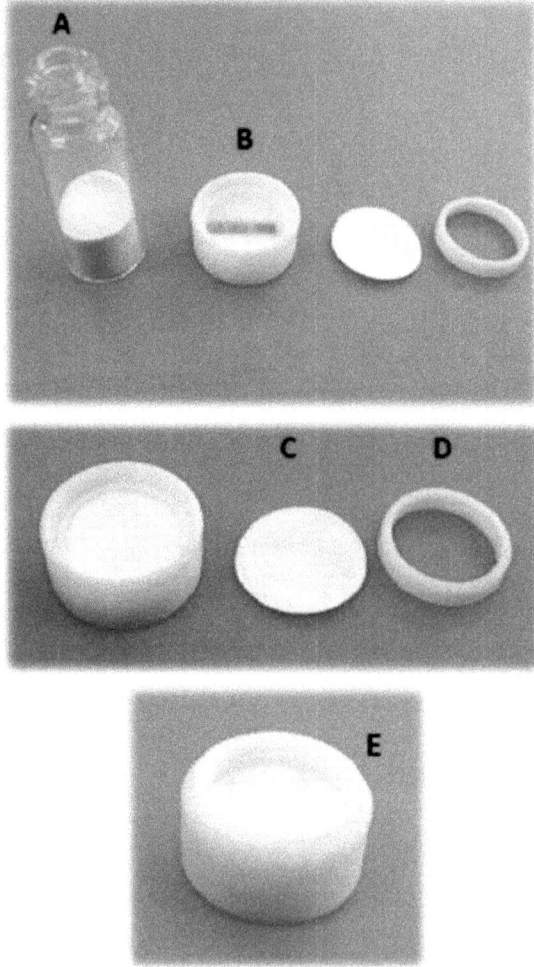

Figure 12. Assembly of rotating sorptive disk extraction (RDSE). Source: [30].

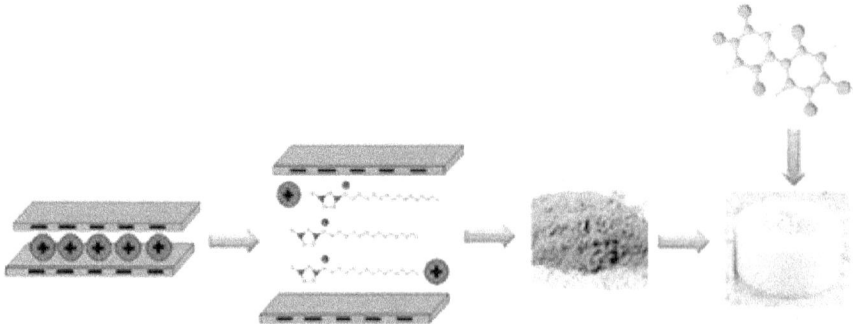

Figure 13. Schematic preparation of new sorbent phase on basis of montmorillonite intercalated with ionic liquids.

Analyte	Matrix	Microextraction technique	Chromatographic system	LoD ng mL^{-1}	LDR ng mL^{-1}	Recovery %	RSD %	Reference
THMs	Drinking water	HF-SBME	GC-μECD	0.017-0.037	10-900	74-91	5.7-10.3	[33]
THMs	Drinking water	HS-SPME	GC-μECD	0.057-0.319	5-200.	74.7-120.9	1.8-11.0	[41]
THMs	Drinking water	HF-LPME	GC-ECD	0.018-0.049	0.88-337.5	80.3-104.2	1.8-3.7	[23]
		HS	GC-MS	0.023-0.102	1.04-230.8	86.3-90.0	6.8-7.8	
HAA	Waste water	EME	HPLC-UV	0.72-40.3 (pg mL^{-1})	5-200	87-106	2.9-6.7	[42]
HAN	Drinking water	DLLME	GC-MS			79-105		[19]
HAA	River and tap water	SDME	GC-MS			82-98		[19]
THMs	Water	SBSE	GC-HRMS	N.R		N.R		[19]
THMs	Tap and recycled waters	HS	GC-μECD	0.09-0.14	0.1-100		2.4-4.3	[43]
HAN,HK	Drinking water	SPME	GC-MS	2-180	0.01-20	N.R.	4-7	[44]
HAA	Drinking water	SBME	GC-μECD		1-100			[45]
THMs	Drinking water	ITEX	GC-MS	1-10 (pg mL^{-1})		90-103	< 10	[25]
THMs	Drinking water	SPME with MMT-IL-AF under liquid desorption	GC-μECD	0.020	2-500	> 75	< 12	This work
PCBs	Drinking water	RDSE	GC-ECD	3-43 (pg mL^{-1})	500-3000	80-86	2-24	[40]
TCS	Drinking water	RDSE	GC-MS	1.8	1000-5000	70		[45]
Parabens	River and Tap waters	RDSE-cork	LC-MS/MS	0.27	0.80-75	80.1-123.9	< 17	[46]
		RDSE-clay		2.0	6-50	82.4-119.9	< 13	
		RDSE-C18		4.2	12.5-100			

LoD: Limit of detection; LDR: Linear dynamic range; RSD: Relative standard deviation.

Table 3. Developed methods for analyzing DBPs (and other halogenated compounds) by using microextraction techniques as sample preparation and greener sorbents.

that was supported onto the top of a rotating disk or as a novel SPME configuration for head space extraction of volatile DBPs (**Figure 14**).

For other side, in 2016, we used the bio sorbents cork and clay for the development of the method for analyzing of four parabens: methyl 4-hydroxybenzoate, ethyl 4-hydroxybenzoate, propyl 4-hydroxybenzoate and isobutyl 4-hydroxybenzoate as the targets compounds because they are widely used as preservatives in daily hygiene products and are associated with the

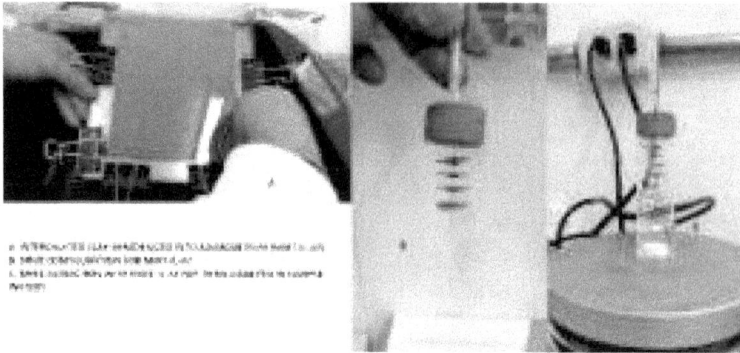

Figure 14. Preparation of the new eco-material and extraction assembly.

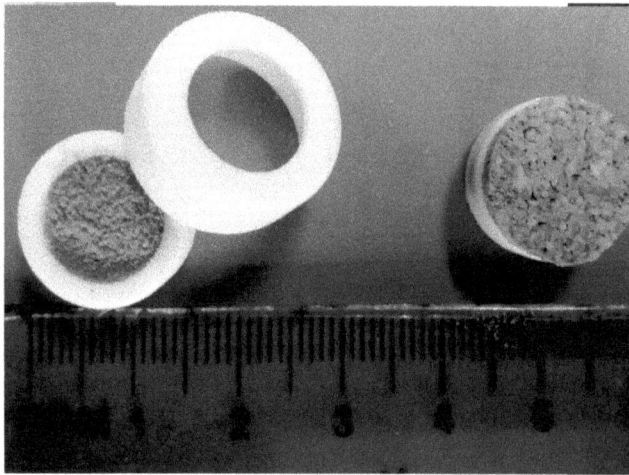

Figure 15. Device used in RDSE.

incidence of cancer. The rotating-disk sorptive extraction (RDSE) was used as supported device for the above mentioned biomaterials (**Figure 15**).

2.10. Sampling and monitoring of aqueous matrices for DBPs analysis

Once reviewed the new microextraction techniques and the possibilities for using greener sorbents, let us present in **Table 3** the different arrangements for the analysis of DPBs by using these new procedure for sample preparation.

3. Conclusions

The existence nowadays over 500 by-products disinfection in low concentrations, by requesting for more sensible and more selectiveness methods of analysis in water samples and all matrices of its whole water's production cycle (wastewater, sludge and surrounded wells samples) and their big direct implications in the public health, is leading to develop new methodologies for their extraction, signal magnification and validate analysis but inspired in the green chemistry ideology. In this sense, the microextraction techniques, a very interesting role until now have been complied, because in the one whole step, they can isolate, preconcentrate and cleanup the target analytes from proved matrix's interferences using less amounts of toxic organic solvents invocating the necessity of automation and with obviously enhancing of its performance and its analytical figures. Some researchers have been pointed that the new trends in the analysis are requesting for developing greener and more selectiveness sorbents/solvents by attaching the high performance of the revised miniaturized methods in this chapter with the advantages of these new eco-materials that are biodegradable materials, has been generated less production of waste, and these composites have a wide natural distribution by assuring the equilibrium of the relationships between the man and its environment.

Acknowledgements

The author is gratefully with the Vicerrectoría de Investigaciones y Postgrados (VIP) of the Caldas University for the financial support during the last 4 years.

Author details

Milton Rosero-Moreano

Address all correspondence to: milton.rosero@ucaldas.edu.co

Universidad de Caldas, Facultad de Ciencias Exactas y Naturales, Departamento de Química, Grupo de Investigación en Cromatografía y Técnicas Afines GICTA, Manizales, Colombia

References

[1] Kokosa JM, Przyjazny A, Jeannot MA. Solvent Microextraction: Theory and Practice. 1st editor. New Jersey: Wiley; 2009. 323 p

[2] Rook JJ. Formation of halforms during chlorination of natural waters. Journal of Water Treatment Examination. 1974;23:234-243

[3] Rosero-Moreano M, Nerín C, Taborda-Ocampo G, Rodríguez-Martínez G. Caracterización química de la materia orgánica natural del río Pasto. Revista de la Academia Colombiana de Ciencias Exactas. 2011;35(136):363-369

[4] Aguirre M. Evaluación de la presencia de subproductos de desinfección en la Planta de Viterbo, Caldas [Master's Thesis]. Manizales: Universidad de Caldas; 2012

[5] Chamorro Bolaños X, Rosero-Moreano M, Enríquez AL. Materia Orgánica y Trihalometanos en Agua para Consumo Humano. 1a ed. Saarbrücken, Deutschland Editorial Académica Española; 2012. ISBN: 978-3659-03818-1

[6]   Bromine and Iodine toxicity [Internet] www.toxnet.com [Available on November 2017]

[7]   Craun GF. Waterborne Diseases in the United States. Boca Raton, FL: CRC Press; 1985

[8]   Craun G. Conference Conclusions, Proc. First International Conference on the Safety of Water Disinfection. Washington, DC: ILSI Press; 1993. 657-667

[9]   Ashbolt NJ. Risk analysis of drinking water microbial contamination versus disinfection by-products (DBPs). Toxicology. 2004;**198**:255-262

[10] Correa-Chacón L, Rosero-Moreano M, Taborda-Ocampo G. Análisis de ácidos haloacéticos en muestras de agua utilizando microextracción de barra de solvente de fibra hueca HF-SBME con derivatización dentro de la membrana. In: Proceedings of the XII Latin American Symposium on Environmental Analytical Chemistry (XII LASEAC Colombia); 23-27 April 2017; Manizales; 69

[11] Guidelines for Drinking Water. WHO; 2016

[12] Rules for THMs in Drinking Water [Internet]. www.epa.gov.co [Available on November 2017]

[13] Normative for Drinking Water in the European Union. Commission of European Union [Internet]. www.eu.com [Available on November 2017]

[14] Epidemiological and Toxicological Studies on Cancer From Drinking Water. IARC [Internet] www.iarc.com.ca [Available on November 2017]

[15] Asensio E, Sanagustín F, Nerín C, Rosero-Moreano M. Improvement of biodegradable biocide's activity of peroxyacetic acid basis using surfactants: Characterization and stability. Journal of Chemistry. 2015:9 p. DOI:DOI 10.1155/2015/150206

[16] Cancho B, Ventura F. Optimization of methods for the determination of DBPs. Global NEST Journal. 2005;**7**:72-94

[17] Thurman EM, Mills MS, Solid-Phase Extraction: Principles and Practice. 1st ed. New York: Wiley; 1998. 344 p

[18] Pastor SJ, Krasner SW, Weinberg HS, Richardson SD. Solid-phase extraction – Gas chromatography/mass spectrometry for the investigation of newly identified disinfection by-products in drinking water. Proceedings of 48th American Society of Mass Spectrometry Conference (ASMS) on Mass Spectrometry, Long Beach, Calif; 2000

[19] Kinani A, Kinani S, Bouchonnet S. Formation and determination of organohalogen by-products in water – Part II. Sample preparation techniques for analytical approaches. Trends in Analytical Chemistry. 2016;**85**:281-294

[20] Rosero-Moreano M. Estudio exploratorio sobre la presencia de materia orgánica natural y subproductos de la desinfección con cloro en la planta potabilizadora de Puerto Mallarino, Cali-Colombia [Mater's Thesis]. Cali: Universidad del Valle; 2004

[21] Rosero-Moreano M, Latorre-Montero J, Torres W, Delgado LG. Buenas Prácticas en la Validacion de Técnicas de Cuantificacion de Orgánicos en el Agua. Caso Sistema de Tratamiento de Agua para Consumo Humano, Puerto Mallarino, Cali-Colombia. In: Proceedings of the International Seminar: Integral Vision in the Improvement of Water Quality (AGUA 2005); 01-04 June 2005; Cali; 12

[22] Richardson SD. The role of GC-MS and LC-MS in the discovery of drinking water disinfection by-products. Journal of Environmental Monitoring. 2002;**4**:1-9

[23] Rosero-Moreano M, Aguirre M, Pezo D, Taborda G, Dussán C, Nerín C. Solventless microextraction techniques for determination of trihalomethanes by gas chromatography in drinking water. Water, Air, and Soil Pollution 2012;**223**:667-678. DOI 10.1007/s11270-011-0891-9

[24] Parinet J, Tabaries S, Coulomb B, Vassalo L, Boudenne JL. Exposure levels to brominated compounds in seawater swimming pools treated with chlorine. Water Research. 2012;**46**: 828-836

[25] Laaks J, Jochmann MA, Schilling B, Schmidt TC. In-tube extraction of volatile organic compounds from aqueous samples: An economical alternative to purge and trap enrichment. Analytical Chemistry. 2010;**82**:7641-7648

[26] Arthur CL, Pawliszyn J. Solid phase microextraction with thermal desorption using fused silica optical fibers. Analytical Chemistry. 1990;**62**(19):2145-2148

[27] Jeannot MA, Cantwell FF. Mass transfer characteristics of solvent extraction into a single drop at the tip of a syringe needle. Analytical Chemistry. 1997;**69**(2):235-239

[28] Baltussen E, Sandra P, David F, Cramers C. Stir bar sorptive extraction (SBSE), a novel extraction technique for aqueous samples: Theory and principles. Journal of Microcolumn Separations. 1999;**11**:737-747

[29] Pedersen-Bjergaard S, Rasmussen E. Liquid-phase microextraction and capillary electrophoresis of acidic drugs. Eletrophoresis. 2000;**21**(3):579-585

[30] Richter P, Leiva C, Choque C, Giordano A, Sepúlveda B. Rotating-disk sorptive extraction of nonylphenol from water samples. Journal of Chromatography A. 2009;**1216**(49): 8598-8602

[31] Maya F, Palomino-Cabello C, Ghani M, Turnes-Palomino G, Cerdà V. Emerging materials for sample preparation, Journal of Separation Science. 2018;**41**:262-287

[32] Fiscal-Ladino JA, Correa-Chacón SL, Ceballos-Loaiza S, de la Ossa-Salcedo A, Taborda-Ocampo G, Nerin C, Rosero-Moreano M. Development of a new liquid phase microextraction method with hollow fiber HF-SBME for the analysis of the organochlorine compounds in water samples by GC-ECD. Journal of Separation Science. 2014;**6**(4): 241-250. http://dx.doi.org/10.4322/sc.2015.009

[33] Correa L, Fiscal JA, Ceballos S, de la Ossa A, Taborda G, Nerin C, Rosero-Moreano M. Hollow-fiber solvent bar microextraction with gas chromatography and electron capture detection determination of disinfection by-products in water samples. Journal of Separation Science. 2015;**38**(22):3945-3953

[34] Zhao RS, Wang X, Sun J, Yuan JP, Wang SS, Wang XK. Temperature-controlled ionic liquid dispersive liquid-phase microextraction for the sensitive determination of triclosan and triclocarban in environmental water samples prior to HPLC-ESI-MS/MS Journal of Separation Science. 2010;**33**:1842-1848. DOI 10.1002/jssc.201000080

[35] Sarafraz Yazdi A, Razavi N, Raouf Yazdinejad S. Separation and determination of amitriptyline and nortriptyline by dispersive liquid–liquid microextraction combined with gas chromatography flame ionization detection. Talanta. 2008;**75**(5):1293-1299

[36] Gerstel. Twister/Stir Bar Sorptive Extraction SBSE [Internet]. 2018. Available from: http://www.gerstel.com/en/twister-stir-bar-sorptive-extraction.htm [Accessed: March 10, 2018]

[37] Gerstel. Extractables & Leachables Medical Implants – A closer look [Internet]. 2018. Available from: http://www.gerstel.com/en/GSW15_Extractables_Leachables.htm [Accessed: March 10, 2018]

[38] Valcárcel M, Cárdenas S, Lucena R. Analytical Microextraction Techniques. 1a ed. Bentham Books. ISBN: 978-1-68108-380-3

[39] Tobiszewski M, Marć M, Gałuszka A, Namieśnik J. Green chemistry metrics with special reference to green analytical chemistry. Molecules. 2015;**20**:10928-10946

[40] Fiscal-Ladino JA, Obando-Ceballos M, Rosero-Moreano M, Montaño DF, Cardona W, Giraldo LF, Richter P. Ionic liquids intercalated in montmorillonite as the sorptive phase for the extraction of low-polarity organic compounds from water by rotating-disk sorptive extraction. Analytica Chimica Acta 2017;**953**:23-31

[41] Aguirre M, Rosero-Moreano M. Optimization of the HS-SPME technique by using response surface methodology for evaluating chlorine disinfection by-products by GC in drinking water. Journal of the Brazilian Chemical Society. 2011;**22**(12):2330-2336

[42] Alhooshani K, Basheer C, Kaur J, Gjelstad A, Rasmussenc KE, Pedersen-Bjergaard S, Kee Lee H. Electromembrane extraction and HPLC analysis of haloacetic acids and aromatic acetic acids in wastewater. Talanta. 2011;**86**:109-113

[43] Alexandrou LD, Meehan BJ, Morrison PD, Jones OAH. A new method for the fast analysis of trihalomethanes in tap and recycled waters using headspace gas chromatography with micro-electron capture detection. International Journal of Environmental Research and Public Health. 2017;**14**(5):527-533

[44] Riazi-Kermani F, Tugulea A-M, Hnatiw J, Niri VH, Pawliszyn J. Application of automated solid-phase microextraction to determine haloacetonitriles, haloketones, and chloropicrin in Canadian drinking water. Water Quality Research Journal. 2013;**48**(1): 85-98. DOI:10.2166/wqrjc.2013.012

[45] Rosero-Moreano M, López-Calvo A, Sánchez-Duque G, Hara E, Taborda-Ocampo G, Richter P, Grassi MT. Ionic liquid intercalated in montmorillonite impregnated agarose film supported on rotating disk sorptive extraction of triclosan in water samples. In: Proceedings of the XXXII Chilean Meeting of Chemistry (XXXII JChQ Chile); 09-12 January 2018; Puerto Varas; 200 p

[46] Vieira C, Mazurkievicz M, Lopez-Calvo AM, Debatin V, Micke GA, Richter P, Rosero-Moreano M, Carasek E. Exploiting green sorbents in rotating-disk sorptive extraction for the determination of parabens by UPLC-ESI/MS/MS. Submitted on Journal of Separation Science A. April 2018

[47] On J, Pyo HS, Myung SW. Effective and sensitive determination of disinfection byproducts in drinking water by DLLME and GC–MS. International Journal of Environmental Analytical Chemistry. Submitted on October 2017

[48] Golfinopoulos SK, Nikolaou AD, Lekkas TD. The occurrence of disinfection by-products in the drinking water of Athens, Greece. Environmental Science and Pollution Research. 2003;**10**(6):368-372

www.ingramcontent.com/pod-product-compliance
Lightning Source LLC
Chambersburg PA
CBHW070156240326
41458CB00127B/5871